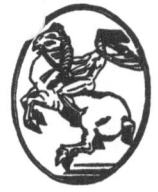

ACTA NEUROCHIRURGICA
SUPPLEMENTUM 24

Advances in Stereotactic and Functional Neurosurgery 2

**Proceedings of the 2ⁿᵈ Meeting
of the European Society for Stereotactic
and Functional Neurosurgery, Madrid 1975**

**Edited by
F. J. Gillingham, E. R. Hitchcock**

SPRINGER-VERLAG
WIEN   NEW YORK

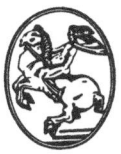

F. JOHN GILLINGHAM

Professor of Neurosurgery, University of Edinburgh,
Western General Hospital and Royal Infirmary, Edinburgh

EDWARD R. HITCHCOCK

Consultant Neurosurgeon, University of Edinburgh,
Western General Hospital and Royal Infirmary, Edinburgh

With 89 Figures

Library of Congress Cataloging in Publication Data.

European Society for Stereotactic and Functional Neurosurgery. Advances in stereotactic and functional neurosurgery. (Acta neurochirurgica: supplementum; 24.) 1. Stereoencephalotomy-Congresses.
2. Cerebral palsy-Surgery-Congresses. 3. Movement disorders-Surgery-Congresses. 4. Pain-Surgery-
Congresses. I. Gillingham, Francis John. II. Hitchcock, Edward Robert. III. Title. IV. Series [DNLM:
1. Neurosurgery-Congresses. 2. Stereotaxic technics-Congresses. 3. Cerebral palsy-Surgery-Congresses.
4. Hyperkinesis-Surgery-Congresses. 5. Pain-Surgery-Congresses. 6. Evoked potentials-Congresses.
7. Neurophysiology-Congresses. W1 AC8661 no. 24/WL368 E89a 1975]. RD594.E85. 1977.
617'.481. 77-22266.

ISBN-13: 978-3-211-81422-2   e-ISBN-13: 978-3-7091-8482-0
DOI: 10.1007/978-3-7091-8482-0

Contents

Section III. Neurophysiology

Section IV. Pain

Section I

Cerebral Palsy and Hyperkinesias

Acta Neurochirurgica, Suppl. 24, 3–10 (1977)
© by Springer-Verlag 1977

Juntendo University School of Medicine, Tokyo, Japan

Experiences of Stereotaxic Surgery on Cerebral Palsy Patients

H. Narabayashi

With 5 Figures

Cerebral palsy or spasticity is a broad term which encompasses a varied aetiology and pathology. The clinical and physiological manifestations are motor, intellectual and emotional.

Patients selected for stereotaxic surgery should be those with motor disturbances only, with normal or, at least, borderline intelligence and with high motivation for recovery even though it involves long-term physiotherapy. Patients with marked or relative feeblemindedness or with severe epileptic signs should not be considered.

Taking those cases mainly with motor disturbances, the type of clinico-physiological features of motor symptoms were analyzed and disclosed as described previously (Narabayashi and Nakamura 1972). One of the most basic features is the increase of muscle tone, which can be demonstrated by the presence of tonic stretch reflexes with passive stretching of muscles, as in parkinsonian rigidity. However the explanation is not so clear and so simple as in Parkinsonism. One of the important differences is found in the distribution of such hypertonicity. In Parkinsonism, muscular hypertonicity is diffuse in agonist, antagonist and related coordinating muscles. But in cerebral palsy there usually exists some imbalance between muscles, resulting in specific postures of the trunk and extremities in each case. For example, spasm of the external rotator muscles at the shoulder joint results in extreme extension and lateral rotation of the arm. Similarly, adduction spasm of the thigh, semiflexion spasm at the knee and inversion of foot are caused by dominant hypertonus of muscles responsible for each of these abnormal postures. Another important difference is that the level of the hypertonus fluctuates in tension-athetoid or remains at a static level, but mixed with spasticity in both spastic and rigid types.

1*

Aetiologically most patients have suffered from cerebral anoxia, either by perinatal or in early infancy when infantile fébrile convulsions are common. In choreoathetosis there is almost no hypertonicity and the conditions is mostly due to severe kernicterus. For these patients there are few indication for surgery since signs of muscular hypertonicity are difficult to detect. Reviewing these, the commonly used classification in cerebral palsy, such as the spastic, rigid, or athetoid type can be interpreted as shown (Fig. 1).

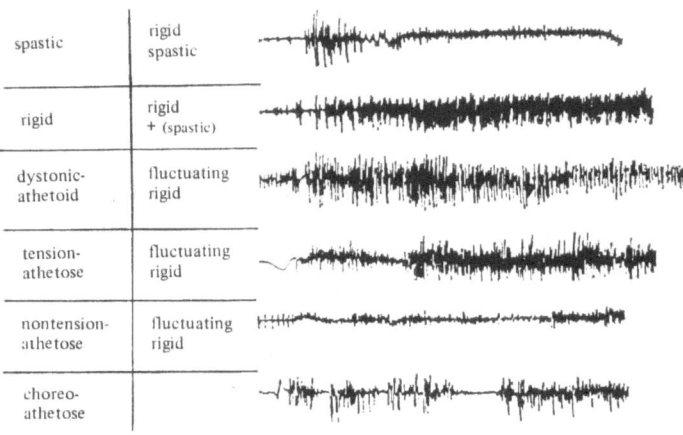

Fig. 1. Pattern of stretch reflexes in different types of cerebral palsy (from Confin. Neurol. *34*, 7—13 [1972], Narabayashi and Nakamura). Except the last group "choreo-athetose", the main dominating feature of muscular contraction in CP cases is rigidity, as shown on the right side of each classified type. The grade and pattern of rigidity and fluctuation of the level of rigidity differs in type

By means of a stereotaxic lesion mainly in the area of the ventral border of the VL and Vim nuclei of the thalamus, hypertonicity is relieved, without any associated weakness or pyramidal signs as in Parkinsonism. In order to overcome the problems of anatomical variation of the child brain from that of the adult brain, when using the atlas physiological monitoring is essential. For example analysis of cortical evoked potentials from thalamic stimulation or analysis of unit activity of thalamic cells.

Changes of external rotator and extensor spasm at the shoulder are shown (Figs. 2 a and b). After improvement of hypertonicity of the external rotator muscles, the arm can be brought down or forward in various degrees which was completely impossible preoperatively.

Active Movement at Shoulder in 28 cases

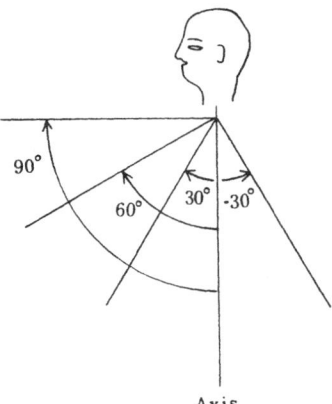

Axis

grade of disturb.	angle of movement	no. of cases
mild	60° — 90°	8 cases
moderate	30° — 60°	6
severe	0 — 30°	3
most severe	-30° — 0	11

a

Fig. 2 a. Indicates the grade of spasm of the external rotator muscle at the shoulder-girdle shown by the range of movements

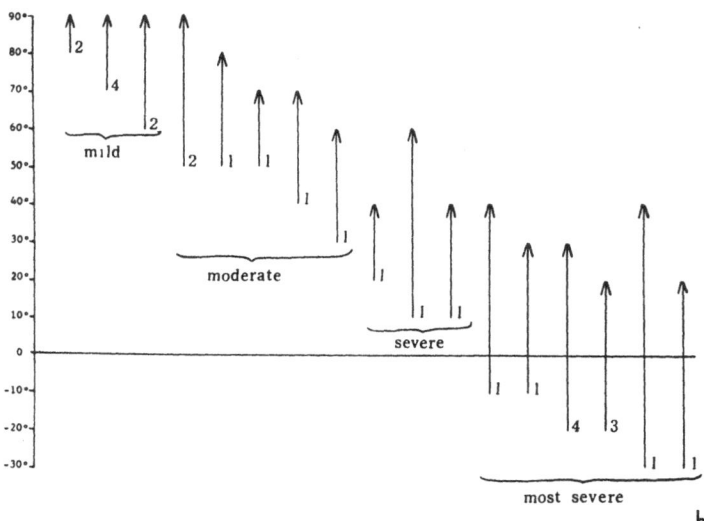

b

Fig. 2 b. Each groups of differing severity are improved by surgery as indicated by an arrow to a wider range of movements. The number is the number of improved cases in the total of 28 cases

When physiotherapy is maintained for long periods such improvement is observed to persist, one example of which (case of right-sided hemispasticity, due to febrile convulsions in childhood) is shown in Fig. 3.

However, the problems after the surgical procedure is quite different from those in Parkinsonism, namely the establishment of voluntary control of movement and posture. I do not intend to

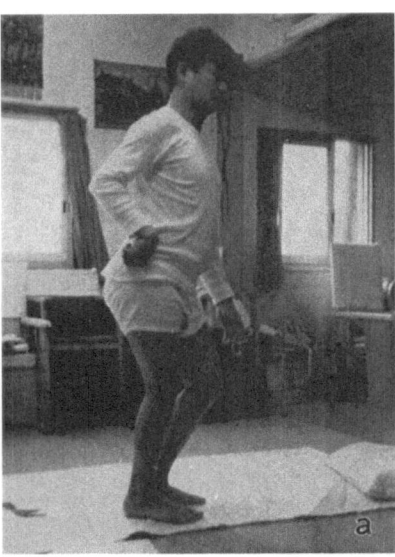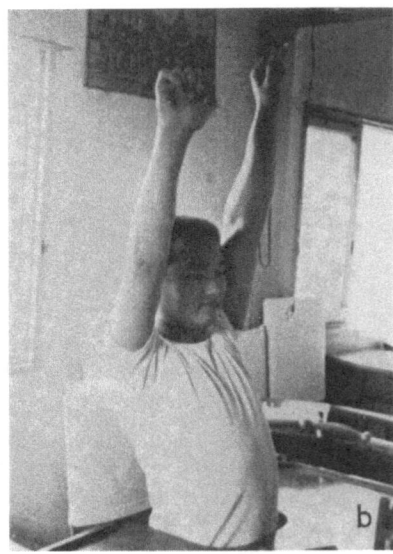

Fig. 3. Twenty-three-year-old boy with right sided spasticity. Preoperatively (a) due to shoulder spasm and freezing, he could not raise his arm at all. There became normal after surgery and about five months postoperative rehabilitation (b). However, note that the right fingers are not significant changed and have maintained a flexed posture

refer to the details of physiotherapy but the basic problem is inhibition of primitive reflexes and encouragement or teaching of the developmental sequences of the movement pattern, especially those in posture of the trunk. Such postoperative physiotherapy follows a *neurodevelopmental approach,* which is commonly known as the Bobath method, although the Bobath technique is mainly for infants or younger children.

In the following, several observations will be described. Fig. 4 is a picture of 11 years old boy, who was severely dystonic and unable to sit or even to sleep supine preoperatively. He is now able

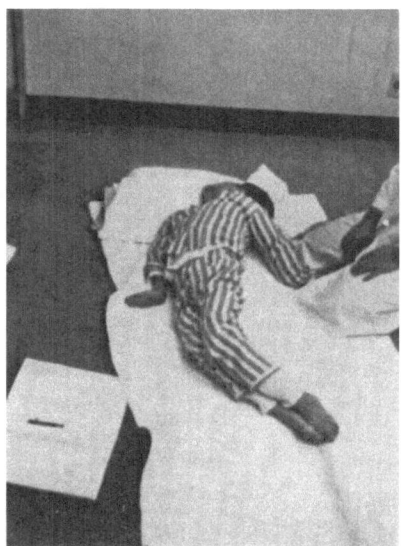
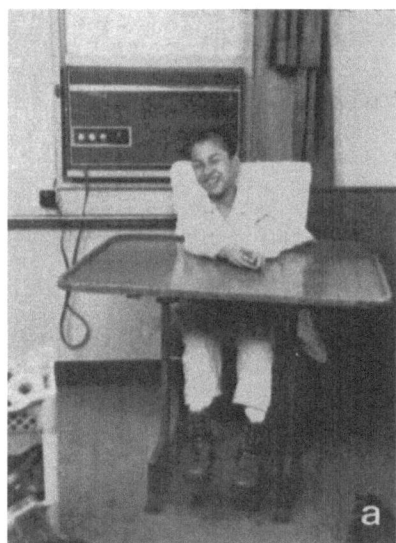
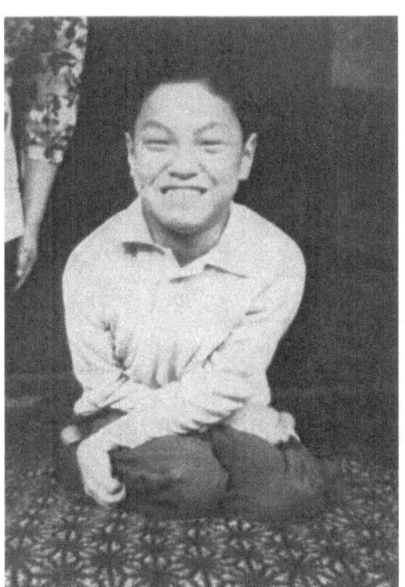
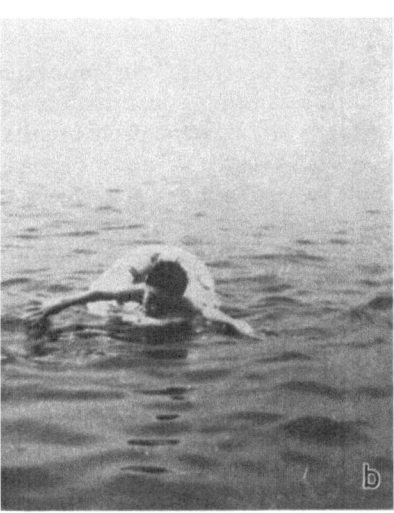

Figs. 4 a and b. Eleven-year-old boy severe dystonic and opisthotonic (pre-operative = left, postoperative = right). Three months after operation (bilat. thalamotomy in two stages with an interval of two months between each) he is able to sit on a chair and in five months he was able to sit alone (4 b, left) and in seven months he could relax and float on water for pleasure (4 b, right)

to sit in a wheelchair and move by himself and use a head type-writer. Another severely dystonic case, also an 11 years old boy (Fig. 5), had torsion of the pelvis and could not sleep or lie supine. After operation he was able to sit by himself and started to attend school.

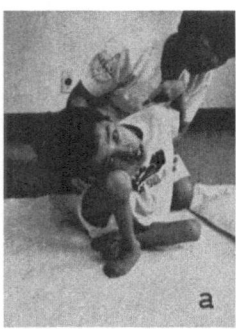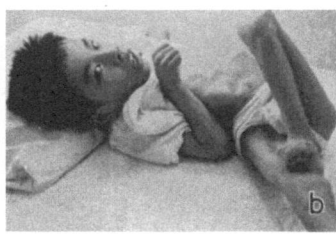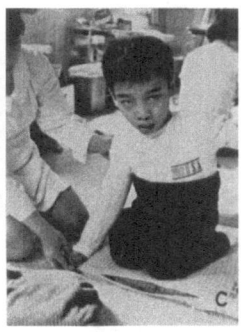

Fig. 5. Eleven-year-old boy with severe torsion of the pelvis and truncal dystonia. One year after left thalamotomy and physiotherapy, he was able to sit up and attend school. a) and b) preoperative, c) one year postoperative

Table 1 present the improvement of speed in some skilled move-ments involving coordination. It seems important to mention that the rate of acceleration is usually + 30% or + 40% compared with preoperatively. It never becomes completely normal, and this may indicate the limits of surgery as regards total relief of muscular hypertonus.

From our experiences over the past twenty-five years the follow-ing can be stated.

When excessive hypertonus producing severe abnormal posture in cerebral palsy is difficult to control or to manage by conservative treatment, stereotaxic thalamotomy is useful as the best means of reduction of such abnormal muscular hypertonus.

The hypertonus usually reaches maximum around early school age and then tends to continue with development, sometimes followed by secondary peripheral changes. When such hypertonus with severe postural disorders has appeared, there is a clearly a limit to conserva-tive management even by the most skilled physiotherapist.

In my experience, bearing in mind the importance of exact clinical assessment of the motor disability and of the psychological and physical problems operation is never indicated below early school age and at the same time operation is contraindicated in adults in whom secondary peripheral changes have occurred.

Table 1. *Improvement in Skill (Speed) in Some Simple Voluntary Movements in ADL*

Movement		Athetoid (12 cases)		Spastic (4 cases)	
		preope.	postope.	preope.	postope.
upper extr.	extension & flexion at elbow (per min.)	33	43 (+10)	63	70 (+7)
	opening & fist making of fingers	53	64 (+11)	18	20 (+2)
	finger touch (thumb & index finger)	110	130 (+20)	impossible	
	picking up the small bars	26	30 (+4)	9	10 (+1)
	adduction & abduction at shoulder	8	14 (+6)	6	10
lower extr.	speed of gait (100m)	72 sec.	54 (+18)	56	40 (-16)
	knee extension & flexion (per min.)	23	31 (+8)	23	30 (+7)

Stereotaxic thalamotomy is a means of making untrainable severe cases of postural abnormality trainable and manageable. Without postoperative long-term physiotherapy, the results would be poor. The effects of operation is not so dramatic as in Parkinsonism but it is still helpful when the indications and type of surgical procedure are carefully worked out.

References

Bleck, E. E. (1975), Locomotor prognosis in cerebral palsy. Develop. Med. Child. Neurol. *17*, 18—25.

Bobath, B. (1971), Abnormal postural reflex activity caused by brain lesions. Published in association with The Chartered Society of Physiotherapy. London: William Heinemann Medical Books Ltd.

Bobath, K. (1966), The motor deficit in patients with cerebral palsy. Clinics in Developmental Medicine, No. 23. Published by the Spastics Society Medical Education and Information Unit in association with William Heinemann Medical Books Ltd.

Crothers, B., Paine, R. S. (1959), The natural history of cerebral palsy. Cambridge, Massachusetts: Harvard University Press.

Denhoff, E., Robinault, I. (1960), Cerebral palsy and related disorders. London: McGraw-Hill.

Fukamachi, A., Ohye, C., Narabayashi, H. (1973), Delineation of the thalamic nuclei with a microelectrode in stereotaxic surgery for parkinsonism and cerebral palsy. J. Neurosurg. *39*, 214—225.

Gornall, P., Hitchcock, E., Kirkland, I. S. (1975), Stereotaxic neurosurgery in the management of cerebral palsy. Develop. Med. Child. Neurol. *17*, 279—286.

Laitinen, L. V. (1965), Short-term results of stereotaxic treatment of infantile cerebral palsy. Confin. Neurol. (Basel) *26*, 258.

Narabayashi, H. (1962), Stereotaxis surgery for athetosis or the spastic state of cerebral palsy. Confin. Neurol. (Basel) *22*, 364—367.

— Shimazu, H., Fujita, Y., Shikiba, S., Nagao, T., Nagahata, M. (1960), Procaine-oil-wax pallidotomy for double athetosis and spastic states in infantile cerebral palsy. Neurology *10*, 61—69.

— Nakamura, R. (1972), Clinical picture of cerebral palsy in neurological understanding. Confin. Neurol. (Basel) *34*, 7—13.

— Nagahata, M., Nagao, T., Shimazu, H. (1965), A new classification of cerebral palsy based upon neurophysiologic considerations. Confin. Neurol. (Basel) *25*, 378—392.

O'Reilly, D. E. (1975), Care of the cerebral palsied: Outcome of the past and needs for the future. Develop. Med. Child. Neurol. *17*, 141—149.

Yoshida, M., Yanagisawa, N., Shimazu, H., Givre, A., Narabayashi, H. (1964), Physiological identification of the thalamic nucleus. Arch. Neurol. *11*, 435—443.

Author's address: H. Narabayashi, M.D., Professor of Neurology, Juntendo University School of Medicine, Tokyo, Japan.

Acta Neurochirurgica, Suppl. 24, 11—14 (1977)

Department for Functional Neurosurgery and Neuronuclear Medicine,
Neurosurgical Clinic of the University of Freiburg i. Br.,
Federal Republic of Germany

Multilocular Lesions in the Therapy of Cerebral Palsy*

F. Mundinger and Chr. Ostertag

Summary

The cerebral pareses occurring in early childhood or produced subsequently by trauma or spontaneous cerebral haemorrhages, present a heterogenous symptomatic picture. In the forefront we find the spastic pareses associated with extrapyramidal motor hyperkinesia (athetosis, dystonia, ballism). 36 C.P.-patients were surveyed from 1–4 years after operative intervention.

It is shown that better results can be obtained when multilocular lesions during a single session in correspondence with the dominant group of symptoms are performed (thalamic and subthalamic target points of the extrapyramidal motor nuclei and dentate nucleus). The results are presented. Continuous physical therapy after the operation and a reasonable intellectual level are essential for improvement.

Key words: Stereotaxis, cerebral palsy, spasticity, extrapyramidal hyperkinesia.

Refinement of stereotactic methods and increasing experience in the selection of target points has led to progress in the therapy of motor dysfunction in cerebral palsy (C.P.) only in recent years [4, 5, 8, 9, 10]. Multilocular lesions, performed in one or more operative sessions enable us to vary the target points as required by the patients dominant symptoms [2, 3, 6].

From our large series 36 C.P.-patients were selected and surveyed from 1 to 4 years after the intervention. In 21 patients the aetiology was perinatal anoxic brain damage; 15 others suffered from traumatic or vascular brain damage, resulting in spasticity with or without involuntary movements. In all cases the dominant symptom was spastic hypertonicity.

Using the computer model of our stereotactic apparatus, we take as reference points various cranial structures in order to calculate by

---

* With support of the Special Research Division, Brain Research and Sensory Physiology, SFB 70, E 2, of the Deutsche Forschungsgemeinschaft, Bad Godesberg, Federal Republic of Germany.

means of our data bank the entrance of the foramen of Monro and the corresponding angle to the target point [7]. We then proceed to a direct puncture of the foramen of Monro and carry out a Dimer-X ventriculogram. (Up to now we have performed 630 Dimer-X ventriculograms without serious incidents.)

The development of lesions is begun first in the zona incerta and the dorsolateral ruber using the side protruding electrode, than in the oral ventral, intermediate and ventro-caudal nuclei (Table 1). Both direction and pathway of the side protruding electrode are predetermined for each patient individually using a special program [1].

Table 1. *Targets Used in Spasticity (36 Patients)*

Target	Number
Zona incerta	31
Pulvinar	19
V.O. Basis	6
V. i m	1
Dentate nucleus	14
Other	3
Σ	74

We than destroy the pulvinar and at an interval of at least one week we lesion the ipsilateral dentate nucleus of the cerebellum.

Clinical and postoperative observations reveal that following subthalamotomy and pulvinarotomy spasticity is reduced contralaterally by 20–30% as a rule before the patients has left the operation table. This effect is improved and stabilized in the following days through additional physical therapy. Coagulation in the pulvinar has a favourable effect on spasticity and hyperkinetic movement even when coagulations in the thalamus and subthalamus and dentate nucleus have not led to satisfactory results. Table 2 gives the results of follow-up examinations up to four years. Good means a lasting improvement of the patients motility after elimination of spasticity. Fair means alleviation of hypertonicity and hyperkinesias under constant additional physical therapy.

During the subsequent months after the intervention, usually not before 3–6 months and after a temporary reduction in motor achievements due to muscular hypotonia the patients show further improvement in co-ordinating movements, in muscular activity, brute force and fine finger movements as well.

A similar clinical improvement is shown in cases where an additional dentatomy has been performed simultaneously. As expected the difference is the greater alleviation of spasticity extrapyramidal motor hyperkinesis contralateral to the subcortical cerebral lesion points and ipsilateral to the dentate lesion as compared to ipsilateral lesion alone.

Complications result from lesions at certain sites. Whereas following cerebral subcortical lesions we had no serious complication, two C.P.-children died of untreatable bronchial pneumonia following bilateral dentatomy. Usually several days of intensive care are

Table 2. *Results in 36 C.P.-Patients*

		good	fair	none	worse
Spasticity only	19	12	3	2	2+
Spasticity and hyperkinesias	17	10	3	2	2

Σ 36 pat.

necessary after bilateral dentatomy since electrolyte derangement can occur through hyperthermia, diabetes insipidus (1 case), hyper- and hypotonia. These complications have induced us to perform the dentatomy in two sessions at an interval of several weeks.

Skilled postoperative physical therapy is of great importance. If there is none available the indication for a stereotactic operation is limited. Our experience shows that the best results are obtained with the Bobath-method possibly in combination with Voitja. Only in cases where it is possible to carry out optimal continuous physical therapy and nursing after the operation, either in hospital, at home or in ambulatory clinics or other centers for spastic patients, can the operation aid the C.P.-patients and improve their capacity for active movement. Similarly a patient's poor mental state limits indications and the quality of the results. Physical therapy is essential in order to develop certain movements and coordination or compensatory active motor function and achievement by elimination of faulty patterns. Certain motor functions must be learned anew or relearned and the capacity to use the trunk, extremities, their interplay and reaction to the milieu of daily life. Stereotactic multilocular lesions can help as an initial step in the treatment of cerebral palsied patients.

References

1. Birg, W., Mundinger, F. (1975), Calculation of the position of a side-protruding electrode tip in stereotactic brain operation using a stereotactic brain operation using a stereotactic with polar coordinates. Acta Neurochir. (Wien) *32*, 83—87.
2. Cooper, I. S., Amin, I., Chandra, R., Waltz, J. M. (1973), A surgical investigation of the clinical physiology of the LP-pulvinar-complex in man. J. neurol. Sci. *18*, 89—110.
3. Heimburger, R. F., Whitlock, C. C. (1965), Stereotaxic destruction of the human dentate nucleus. Confin. Neurol. (Basel) *26*, 346—358.
4. Laitinen, L. V. (1965), Short-term results of stereotaxic treatment for infantile cerebral palsy. Confin. Neurol. (Basel) *26*, 258—263.
5. Mundinger, F. (1968), Stereotaktische Eingriffe (extrapyramidale Bewegungsstörungen). In: Chirurgie des Gehirns und Rückenmarks im Kindes- und Jugendalter (Bushe, Glees, eds.), pp. 1011—1067. Stuttgart: Hippokrates.
6. Mundinger, F. (1975), Stereotaktische Operationen am Gehirn. Stuttgart: Hippokrates.
7. Mundinger, F., Reinke, M.-A., Hoefer, Th., Birg, W. (1975), Determination of intra-cerebral structures using osseous reference points for computer-aided stereotactic operations. Appl. Neurophysiol. *38*, 3—22.
8. Mundinger, F., Riechert, T., Disselhoff, J. (1970), Long term results of stereotaxic operations on extrapyramidal hyperkinesia (excluding parkinsonism). Confin. Neurol. (Basel) *32*, 71—78.
9. Narabayashi, H. (1962), Stereotaxic surgery for athetosis or the spastic state of cerebral palsy. Confin. Neurol. (Basel) *22*, 364—367.
10. Siegfried, J. (1973), Methods and results in hyperkinesia and hypertonicity in Recent Progress in Neurol. Surgery (Sano, K., Ishii, S., Le Vay, D., eds.). Proc. of the Symposia of the Fifth International Congress of Neurol. Surgery, Tokyo, October 7–13, 1973.

Authors' address: Prof. F. Mundinger and Dr. Chr. Ostertag, Department for Functional Neurosurgery and Neuronuclear Medicine of the Neurosurgical Clinic of the University of Freiburg i. Br., D-7800 Freiburg i. Br., Federal Republic of Germany.

Acta Neurochirurgica, Suppl. 24, 15—20 (1977)

Department of Surgical Neurology, University of Edinburgh, Scotland

Stereotactic Lesions of the Pulvinar for Hypertonus and Dyskinesias

F. J. Gillingham, E. G. Walsh, and L. F. Zegada

With 2 Figures

This paper is concerned with clinical neurophysiological and histochemical correlative studies on the effect of lesions of the superior pulvinar in the course of treatment of hypertonus and some of the dyskinesias. We have in fact a twenty year study of the superior pulvinar but the first seventeen years of this were accidental. The posterior 15 mm parasagittal track which Guiot and Gillingham decided to use from 1955 led us through the superior part of the pulvinar en route for the areas of v.o.p. and v.o.a. or the thalamus, capsule and pallidum. Nevertheless we do have records to which we can look back with some interest although in the earlier cases accuracy of target siting is inevitably in question before the routine use of depth microelectrode recording in 1963. After crossing the posterior horn of the lateral ventricle the microelectrode began immediately to record cell activity after piercing the ependyma overlying the pulvinar. There was a distinctive pattern of amplitude which was relatively lower than that of the sensory relay nucleus lying anterior to it (Fig. 1). Entering the sensory relay nucleus led to a sudden rise of amplitude which was immediately shown both on the oscillograph but even better from the loudspeaker on auditory monitoring. Within a millimetre evoked responses were obtained from the hand, fingers or face, usually at first of the pressure or joint displacement type. Thus with depth microelectrode recording the extent of the pulvinar can be clearly defined. This is important for two reasons. Firstly, accurate anatomical and physiological correlation is not always possible otherwise and secondly, we found that the average length of the superior pulvinar in the sagittal plane at 15 mm from the mid-line in twelve consecutive cases was 5.83 mm. If the average sagittal dimension of the therapeutic lesion is 5 mm then obviously most of

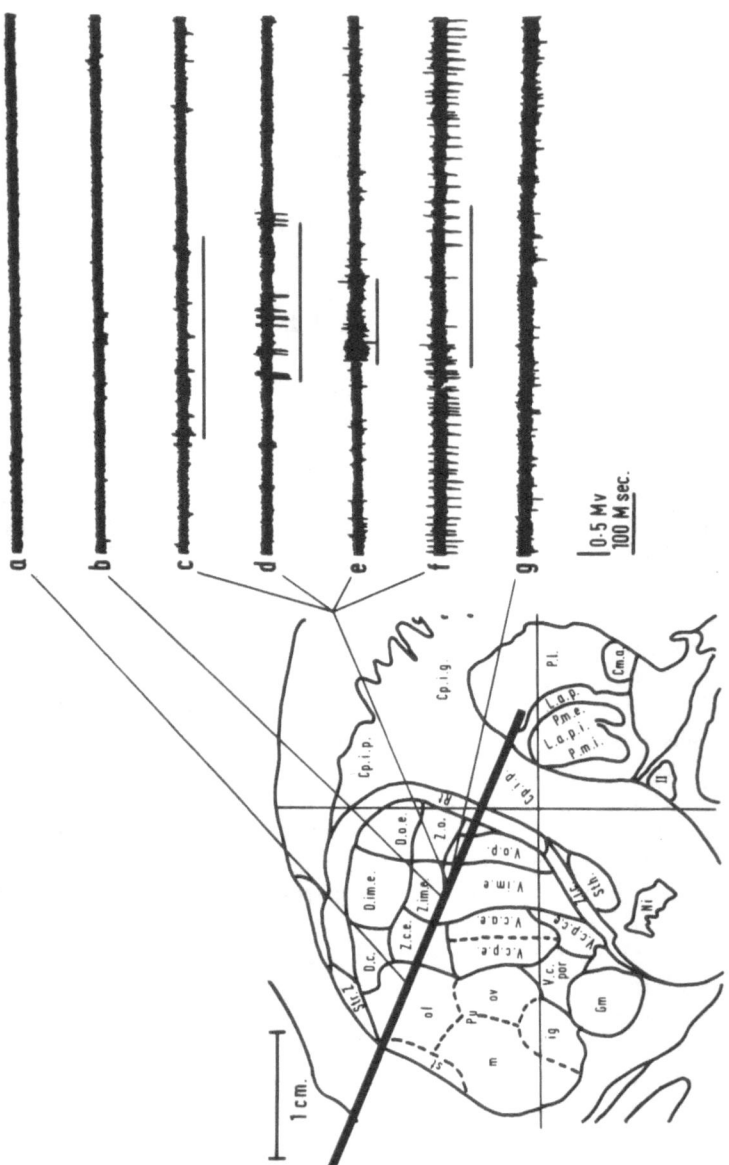

Fig. 1. Depth Microelectrode Recording in the human thalamus using a postero-anterior track 15 mm from the midline

the superior pulvinar is being destroyed. This is important to know because in the past claims were made of specific destruction of nuclei, e.g., the v.o.p. of the thalamus by a lesion larger than the nucleus itself and other areas must inevitably have been involved. Being over-specific is as dangerous as being too vague and in the taking of biopsies it is important to know from which part of a nucleus they have come.

Table 1. *Results of Pulvinar Lesions for the Control of Hypertonus and Dyskinesia*

RESULT

NAME	HYPERTONUS		TREMOR		DYSKINESIA	
	PRE-OP	POST-OP	PRE-OP	POST-OP	PRE-OP	POST-OP
P.C.	++++	+			++++	+
J.W.			+++	+		
R.S.			++++	+		
C.C.	++++	+			++++	+
S.D.	++++					
V.L.			++++	0		
D.C.	++++	0				
S.D.	++++	+				
L.G.	+++	0	+++	0		
N.G.			+++	+		
M.F.					+++	

During these studies of depth electrode recording published in 1964 (Gaze *et al.*) we also observed in Parkinsonian patients spontaneous rhythmical activity, synchronous with tremor but not evoked and only from thalamic nuclei. These findings were occasional and difficult to elicit in every patient but were found only in the pulvinar, v.o.p., v.o.a. and reticular nuclei at 3–5 mm above the AC/PC plane. The explanation still remains elusive.

Stimulation studies of the pulvinar have only been carried out routinely in the past three years using a monopolar electrode because a bipolar concentric electrode with a 1 mm interelectrode distance was less consistent. In the pulvinar no clinical response occurred except at the higher thresholds of stimulation (10 v. at 50 cycles) and it could be argued that such motor or sensory responses were the result of spread. Studies of speech were routinely carried out with the speech therapist and tape recording made before and during the operation under strict local anaesthesia. We could not confirm the observation that stimulation of the pulvinar at least in its superior part leads to arrest of speech or indeed to any other change of speech for the worse, neither in the dominant nor in the non-dominant hemisphere. In one patient with severe intention tremor from multiple sclerosis, dysarthria improved as the lesion was made but presumably as a result of improved co-ordination of speech from restored motor function. However, we did observe cessation of speech in all patients when the threshold of stimulation was high but this always occurred in association with motor or sensory phenomena which distracted the patient. Control studies on normal subjects with unexpected noxious stimulation of the skin caused similar cessation of speech from distraction, as one might expect, and tape recordings of these studies have been made. One or two of the volunteer normal controls succeeded in speaking through the period of stimulation, as indeed did some of the patients when asked to do so, but there was always an alteration of pitch and amplitude.

Previous stimulation studies of the thalamus over the first seventeen years show that most motor, sensory or speech phenomena occur outside the pulvinar and certainly none of our eleven patients with deliberate pulvinar lesions at this level showed any side effects as indicated by Brown *et al.* (1971). Speech disturbances from lesions at other sites have been described by us elsewhere (Hermann *et al.* 1966).

The effects of pulvinar lesions at the superior level on the reduction of hypertonus and involuntary movements in eleven patients over three years are shown (Table 1 and Fig. 2). The method of objective measurement of tone and tremor with "torque induced motion" used by Walsh and Gillingham has been described elsewhere (Gillingham *et al.* 1973), and was used pre-, inter- and postoperatively in each case. When objective measurement showed that reduction of tone or involuntary movements were incompletely reduced by the pulvinar lesion, additional lesions were made in the v.o.p. and v.o.a. areas of the thalamus by advancing the electrode anteriorly. In the fourth patient (C. C.) with dystonia a lesion in the pallidum was also necessary. You see therefore that at this level in the superior pulvinar (a relatively small lesion of 6 × 5 × 5 mm) there was complete reduction of symptoms with a pulvinar lesion alone in only two patients and both of these were patients with Parkinsonian tremor. One of these showed some minor recurrence a few weeks later and may require a further lesion. The ninth patient with multiple sclerosis and combined lesions, although satisfactorily relieved of bilateral intention tremor, showed some mild recurrence within a few days but was nevertheless satisfactorily rehabilitated without further surgery.

Our experience suggests therefore that small lesions of the superior pulvinar may modify the pathological syndromes of hypertonus and dyskinesia satisfactorily and certainly without any defined side effects. Here lies its attraction when bilateral lesions are required. Longer follow-up will show whether the effect will be sustained or whether more extensive lesions will be required. More recent experi-

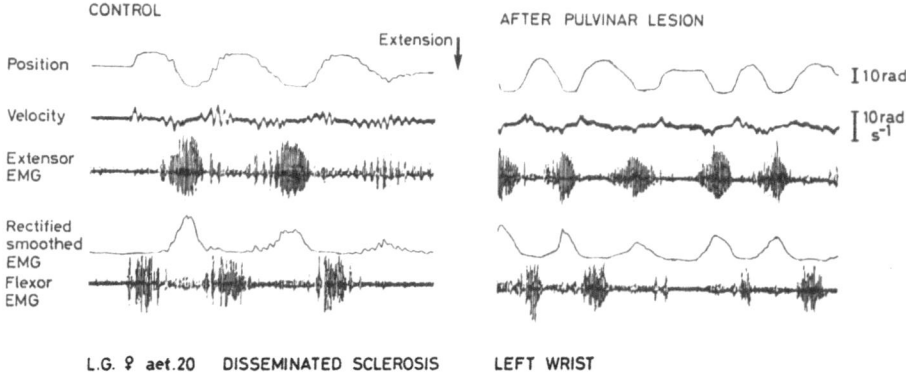

Fig. 2. Monitoring of muscle tonus before and after a stereotactic lesion of the pulvinar

ence suggests that involuntary movements may be as effectively controlled as hypertonus but by larger lesions. The effects would seem to bear a relation, as yet undefined, to the functions of the postural system. This is in accord with Cooper *et al.* (1973) in his observations of lesions of the posterolateral complex of the pulvinar.

Finally in the past two years six patients have had 25 mg biopsies taken from the planned target sites for neurochemical studies. This work was carried out in conjunction with the Medical Research Council Brain Metabolism Unit by Drs. Emerson and Joseph comparing enzyme and amino acid levels and is to be published separately.

References

Brown, J. W., Riklan, M., Waltz, J. M., Jackson, S., Cooper, I. S. (1971), Preliminary studies of language and cognition following surgical lesions of the pulvinar in man. Int. J. Neurol. *8*, 276—296.

Cooper, I. S., Amin, I., Chandra, R., Waltz, J. M. (1973), A surgical investigation of the clinical physiology of the LP-pulvinar complex in man. J. Neurol. Sci. *18*, 89—110.

Gaze, R. M., Gillingham, F. J., Kalyanaraman, S., Porter, R. W., Donaldson, A. A., Donaldson, I. M. L. (1964), Microelectrode recordings from the human thalamus. Brain *87*, 691—706.

Gillingham, F. J., Tsukamoto, Y., Walsh, E. G. (1973), Treatment of rigidity. In: Parkinson's Disease (Siegfried, J., ed.), Vol. 1: Lead of Statement, pp. 94—114. Bern-Stuttgart-Vienna: H. Huber.
Hermann, K., Turner, J. W., Gillingham, F. J., Gaze, R. M. (1966), The effects of destructive lesions and stimulation of the basal ganglia on speech mechanisms. Confin. Neurol. (Basel) 27, 197—207.

Authors' addresses: Prof. F. J. Gillingham, Department of Surgical Neurology, The Royal Infirmary, Lauriston Place, Edinburgh EH3 9YW, Scotland, E. G. Walsh, M.D., Department of Physiology, University of Edinburgh, Scotland, L. F. Zegada, M.D., P. Box 2903, La Paz, Bolivia, South America.

Acta Neurochirurgica, Suppl. 24, 21—26 (1977)

Department of Neurosurgery and its Research Laboratory of Clinical Stereotaxy,
Medical School of Comenius University, Bratislava, ČSSR

Combined Transtentorial Dentatotomy With Pulvinarotomy in Cerebral Palsy

M. Galanda, P. Nádvorník, and M. Šramka

With 1 Figure

Summary

For frequently associated spasticity with involuntary movements in cerebral palsy operations on cerebellar nuclei or on the pulvinar of the thalamus are recommended.

We combined both approaches in 45 patients. The combination was possible after experiences with transtentorial dentatotomy, in which the electrodes are introduced into the deep structures of the cerebellum from a burr-hole on the lambdoid suture. The same lambdoid approach may equally well be applied for introducing electrodes into the pulvinar of the thalamus. The lesion in the pulvinar may moreover be combined with the target in the centrum medianum or in the nuclei VIM-VCP or VOP. Lesions are always asymmetric and multilocular. Their influence on the clinical picture is quite favourable.

The clinical picture in cerebral palsy in children is different from that in adults and therefore they require more complicated stereotactic management. The variability of clinical manifestations are mainly dependent on the time that the brain was damaged, that is during the period when motor activity had not yet come under the control of the cerebral cortex. The subcortical structures of children are more capable of participating in motor organization than in adults. Apart from this, brain lesions in children may be more extensive and numerous than in adults and yet are still compatible with life. Stereotactic treatment can therefore, be applied in children with complicated pathological movements, frequently quite different from each other, although substantially, the pyramidal and extrapyramidal systems will be afflicted.

We had the opportunity of treating 45 patients from 2 to 40 years old, but the majority of them were in the first decade of life. Patients were arranged in several groups (Table 1). Surgical treatment is indicated by individual symptoms or their combinations (Table 2). In our patients, the aims were to improve limb function and daily living.

Table 1. *Syndromological Groups of the Patients*

Diplegia	8
Quadruparesis	5
Hemiplegia	2
Choreoathetosis (double, hemisyndrom)	24
Atypical dyskinesis	6
	45

Table 2. *Symptoms of Cerebral Palsy (in 45 Patients)*

A. Muscular hypertonicity	
spasticity	36
(pure) rigidity	0
rigidospasticity	6
B. Involuntary movements	
athetosis	18
dystonia (of body and/or neck)	3
chorea	6
ballismus	2
intention tremor	1
C. Dependency on emotional state	28
D. Epilepsy	6
E. Mental retardation	26
F. Speech difficulty	31

In the course of the first stage of our approach to cerebral palsy we were supported by our experience with dentatotomy which is carried out by means of a transtentorial approach through the non-dominant hemisphere, usually in the right parieto-occipital region (Nádvorník 1972).

The lesion was made in the ventrolateral part of nucleus dentatus with coordinates 3 mm behind F (fastigium), 3 mm below F, 17 mm laterally from the mid-line. The somatotopical organization of the nucleus was exploited. According to our experience, extremities clinically more afflicted show an earlier response to stimulation under the same technical conditions. The lower threshold of response of appropriate nervous structures is probably the explanation. Co-agulation of the chosen target immediately leads to a marked decrease of muscle tension and similarly improves speech. Long follow-up allows us to assume that the benefits of surgical treatment may be

Table 3. *Strategy of Surgery and Results*

Targets	Improvement		None	
	very good	slight		
Nc. dentatus unilat.			1	1
Nc. dentatus bilat.	3	10	3	16
Nc. dentatus bilat. + pulvinar	4	3		7
Nc. dentatus bilat. + pulvinar + centrum medianum	1	2		3
Nc. dentatus bilat. + pulvinar + VIM-VCP	2			2
Nc. dentatus bilat. + VIM-VCP			1	1
Nc. dentatus unilat. + VIM-VCP + VOAP	1			1
Nc. dentatus bilat. + VOAP	1			1
Pulvinar		3		3
Pulvinar + centrum medianum	1	1		2
Pulvinar + VIM-VCP	1	1		2
VIM-VCP	2	1	1	4
VIM-VCP + VOAP	1			1
VOAP			1	1
	17 (38%)	21	7	45

diminished if postoperative rehabilitation has been unsystematic, incorrect or even lacking. A more lasting result following surgery is shown mostly in antigravity muscles thus improving the postural mechanisms of the body. The final benefits of surgery may also be affected by the age of the patient.

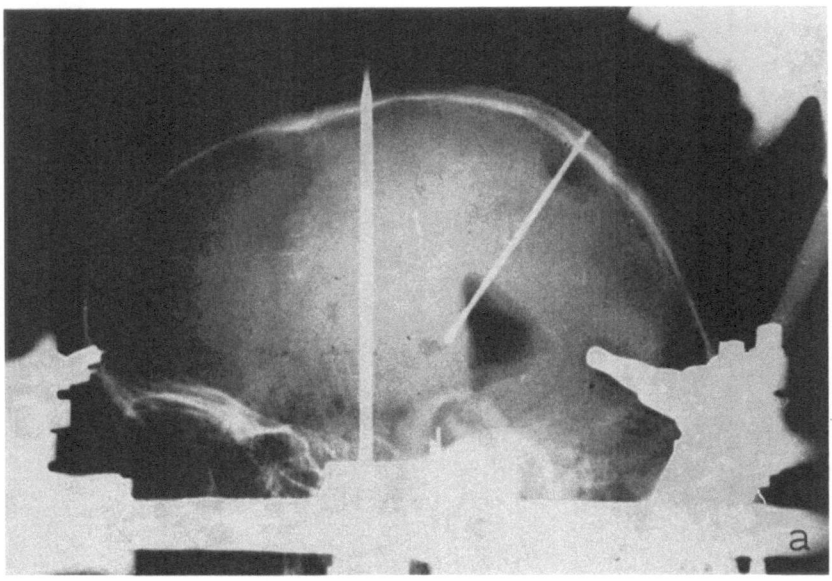

Fig. 1 a

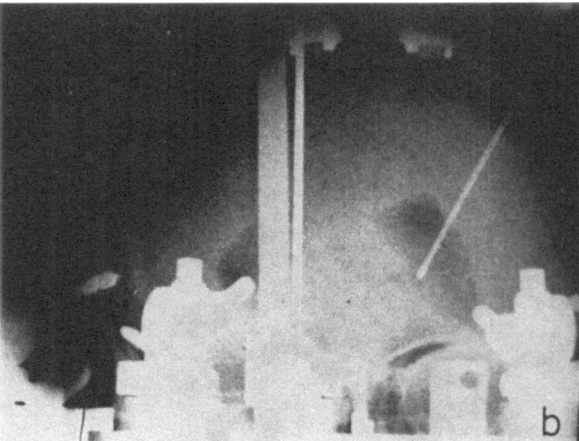

Fig. 1 b

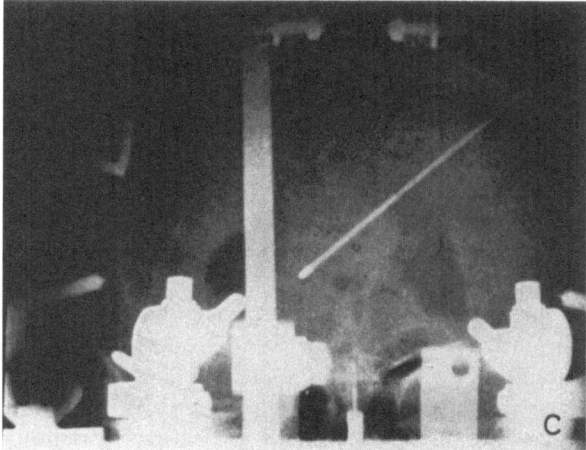

Fig. 1 c

Fig. 1. X-ray control of electrode position in the pulvinar. a) Lateral view,
b) postero-anterior view, homolateral approach, c) transcallosal approach

According to our experience, dentatotomy itself is not quite
sufficient for the adequate treatment of complicated involuntary
movements, and that is why we have mostly combined it with other
targets. The second most frequent target of stereotactic surgery was
the pulvinar. The coordinates we chose for medial pulvinarotomy
were 4 mm behind PC, 4 mm above AC-PC, 12 mm lateral, for lateral
pulvinarotomy 4 mm behind PC, 4 mm above AC-PC, 16 mm
laterally and for LP-complex 10 mm above AC-PC, 14 mm
laterally (Cooper 1972). Using electro-physiological methods of
stimulation responses appears in the contralateral extremities also
reduction of involuntary movement dependent upon the influence of
the hypertonic muscles of the appropriate extremity. Sometimes, the
response is not a very pronounced one, or is absent. However, the
immediate surgical result is quite distinct. The dyskinesis is markedly
suppressed, increased muscle tone decreases and more normal voluntary control occurs.

Later results are much more dependent on rehabilitation, in
which it is necessary to train new movement patterns and thus
replace the abnormal pattern following pulvinarotomy. In the
approach to the pulvinar combined with dentatotomy a burr-hole in
the parieto-occipital region was made. This approach was elaborated
in detail on models and it proved to be a safe one. From a single
burr-hole the contralateral pulvinar may also be approached through

the corpus callosum (Fig. 1). The third structure used for surgery of cerebral palsy is the classical target according to Cooper (1969), *i.e.*, VIM-VCP nuclei thalami. It proved to be useful in patients in whom spasticity is associated with marked rigidity, *i.e.*, in cases of rigidospasticity, and the patient with some involuntary movements. We preferred destruction of these targets in patients in whom involuntary dyskinesias are intensified by intentional movement. We only changed the depth of the electrode in approaching the target and made the lesion on the same trajectory as the pulvinar, *i.e.*, from the occipital approach (lambdoid).

The fourth target used was the centre median of the thalamus (Ramamurthi 1973). It seems to be useful for patients in whom emotional stress markedly increased and intensified the play of involuntary movements. This target may also be reached by the lambdoid approach on a convenient trajectory common with that for the pulvinar.

The last two target areas may also be destroyed by a single large lesion. In combined procedures on the thalamus, the lesion has to spare important nuclei between the two targets. We can achieve this by continuous stimulation determining the region of these nuclei as well as the internal capsule.

Each target is destroyed successively or simultaneously in various combinations to obtain the best results possible for the individual patient (Table 3).

From the lambdoid approach and introducing the electrode through the medial planes of the brain to the contralateral hemisphere, the complications of bilateral surgery are prevented by the creation of asymmetrical lesions. We did not meet with any complications but in one patient, no perceptible benefit was found.

References

Cooper, I. S. (1969), Involuntary movement disorders, p. 423. New York: Hoeber.
— Amin, I., Chandra, R., Waltz, J. M. (1973), A surgical investigation of the clinical physiology of the LP-pulvinar complex in man. J. neurol. Sci. *18*, 89—110.
Nádvorník, P., Šramka, M., Lisý, L., Sviča, I. (1972), Experiences with dentatotomy. Confin. Neurol. (Basel) *34*, 320—324.
Ramamurthi, B. (1973), Central median lesions. An analysis of indications and results in 105 cases. In Sixth Symposium of the International Society for Research in Stereoencephalotomy. Vol. II, p. 16. Tokyo: Abstracts.

Authors' address: MUDr. M. Galanda, Prof. MUDr. P. Nádvorník, and MUDr. M. Šramka, Department of Neurosurgery and its Research Laboratory of Clinical Stereotaxy, Medical School of Comenius University, Bratislava, ČSSR.

Acta Neurochirurgica, Suppl. 24, 27–39 (1977)
© by Springer-Verlag 1977

Neurosurgical Institute of the University of Rome, Rome, Italy

Neurosurgical Treatment of Spasticity and Dyskinesias

B. Guidetti and B. Fraioli

Summary

122 Patients suffering from spasticity and/or dyskinesias underwent a total of 171 operations: 88 stereotactic dentatolyses, 24 posterior partial rootlet section D_{12}-S_1 or L_1-S_1, 16 posterior partial root section D_{12}-S_1 or L_1-S_1, 16 posterior cervical rhizotomies, 21 stereotactic pulvinolyses, 6 stereotactic associated V.L. thalamolysis and pulvinolysis. Results and indications are discussed.

Key words: Different types of spasticity, dystonia, dystonic-athetoid syndromes, choreoathetosis, posterior partial rootlet section, posterior partial root section, posterior cervical rhizotomy, stereotactic dentatolysis, stereotactic pulvinolysis, stereotactic associated V.L. thalamolysis and pulvinolysis.

Clinical Aspects

In our experience we noticed that, while the present clinical classifications of dystonic and choreoathetoid syndromes are sufficient to indicate a particular operation, in the field of spasticity more precise clinical definitions are necessary. That is we are convinced that is not sufficient to define a patient as simply "spastic". In fact there are patients who show spastic disorders only in voluntary movements, other patients who show them in postural conditions, without an increase of them in voluntary movements, and yet more patients who show spastic disorders in postural conditions, but more evident in voluntary movements.

For these reasons, we distinguish, respectively, "phasic spasticity", "tonic spasticity" and "mixed spasticity" [3].

It is opportune to note that this classification derives more from the evaluation of the results of the operations than from a theoretical concept.

Stereotactic Dentatolysis

Between October 1970 and October 1973, 47 dyskinetic patients were operated on.

In 41 patients the operation was carried out bilaterally and in all these cases, except 4, the procedure was performed in one stage. In only 6 patients was the operation unilateral.

The operations were performed on 44 patients under general anaesthesia using endotracheal intubation and on 3 under neurolepto-analgesia.

In all cases pneumoencephalography by the lumbar route was carried out to visualize the 4th ventricle and a Riechert's stereotaxic apparatus, partially modified [8], was used.

According to Nashold and Slaughter's stereotactic coordinates [13], in 4 patients 7 lesions concerning both the ventrolateral and ventro-intermediate part of the dentate nucleus were performed; in 6, on the other hand, 12 lesions concerning both the dorsolateral and dorso-intermediate part were performed; while in 37 patients 69 lesions concerning the entire lateral and intermediate parts of the nucleus were performed. This last type of lesion, bilaterally performed in one stage, gave the best functional results. It extends with respect to the apex of 4th ventricle approximately from 6 mm anterior to 10 mm posterior and from 2 mm superior to 12 mm inferior, on the lateral projections of the radiograms. It is oriented along the long axis of the nucleus and on the frontal plane extends from 10 to 23 mm from the mid-line.

As shown in Table 1, only two out of 18 patients suffering from dystonic or dystonic-athetoid syndromes had unsatisfactory results, and it should be noticed that both these patients were suffering from an evolutive dyskinetic syndrome, that is from dystonia musculorum deformans. In the other patients, on the contrary, suffering from outcomes of infantile cerebral palsy, we observed moderate and also marked improvements of the clinical syndrome. Axial dystonia, and especially dystonia of the trunk, was the best influenced symptom. In particular one patient acquired after the operation not only a correct sitting position, but also an independent walking.

The improvement of dystonic-athetoid symptoms was more noticeable in the upper rather than the lower limbs. In particular 3 patients were able, after the operation, to open and close their hands easily—this was impossible before.

In only 2 of 5 patients affected by choreoathetosis was it observed that a significant improvement of symptomatology occurred and this concerned especially the athetoid component.

In infantile spastic hemiplegia, useful results were observed in 5 of 7 patients operated on. In particular, favourable results were obtained in three patients operated on bilaterally.

In infantile spastic diplegia we observed favourable results in

7 patients who showed spasticity of a mode rate degree, while in 4 other patients suffering from serious spasticity the results were not satisfactory.

None of 6 patients affected by infantile spastic quadriplegia really improved after the operation.

Table 1. *Results of 88 Stereotactic Dentatolyses in 47 Patients*

Condition	Type of spasticity	Markedly improved	Improved	Slightly improved	Unchanged	Totals
Infantile dystonia		2	6			8
Dystonia mus-colorum deformans					2	2
Choreoathetosis			2	2	1	5
Dystonic-athetoid infantile syndromes		2	6			8
Infantile spastic hemiplegia	mixed	1	4	1	1	7
Infantile cerebral diplegia	phasic		2			2
	tonic		1	2		3
	mixed		4	2		6
Infantile cerebral quadriplegia	tonic				3	3
	mixed			1	2	3
Totals		5	25	8	9	47

Neurological complications were only temporary and included: horizontal nystagmus associated with fine upper limb tremor in one case lasting some weeks, and complete absence of speech in two cases for 1 month and 3 months, respectively. Afterwards these two patients had the same speech as they had before the operation.

It is worth reporting that in the patient presenting with nystagmus and tremor, bilateral stereotactic dentatolysis partially involved the medial parts of the nuclei, that is the medial limit of the presumed lesion was 7–8 mm from the mid-line. In another patient, suffering from infantile spastic diplegia and affected by coarse horizontal nystagmus (on right lateral gaze only) bilateral lesions of the entire lateral and intermediate parts of the dentate nuclei in one stage, completely abolished this symptom, which remained abolished two years from the time of operation.

According to previous observations [9, 10, 14, 16] our experience demonstrates then that stereotactic dentatolysis favourably influences dystonic and dystonic-athetoid syndromes.

As regards spastic syndromes, results were less favourable and appeared to be related to the type of clinical syndrome and to the degree of spasticity. In fact the operation, not effective in infantile spastic quadriplegia, was useful only in infantile spastic hemiplegia, only if performed bilaterally, and also in infantile spastic diplegia. Moreover the reduction of spasticity was in general of moderate degree, so that satisfactory functional results were not obtained in serious spastic syndromes. According to our classification we have observed that the operation of dentatolysis can influence both "phasic" and "tonic" spasticity, but we do not believe that "tonic" spastic syndromes benefit satisfactorily. In fact these syndromes generally show serious spasticity which responds more consistently from partial posterior spinal nerve root and rootlet section [7, 5].

Posterior Partial Root Section (Rhizotomy)

Between March 1972 and April 1973, 16 spastic patients were operated on according to the Foerster method [2], technically modified by Gros *et al.* [7]; that is section of all the rootlets which constitute the posterior roots, except one on every root.

In 7 patients, posterior partial rhizotomy was performed from D_{12} to S_1, while in 9 from L_1 to S_1. In all cases the operation was performed bilaterally.

The patients' ages ranged from 6 to 20 years and in all, except one, in whom the clinical syndrome was caused by a trauma of the spinal cord, the etiology of the spastic syndrome was concerned with the usual perinatal pathology.

The clinical picture was stable in all cases. Infantile spastic quadriplegia was the pattern in 7 patients, infantile spastic diplegia in an other 7, post-traumatic spastic paraplegia in 1 and a spastic-dystonic syndrome in one patient. This last had been previously operated on by stereotaxic dentatolysis, with only slight benefit with regard to the spastic component of the syndrome.

In all cases the spastic syndrome was severe and none of the patients could stand unaided.

The functional results obtained in these patients are reported in Table 2. As shown, 12 out of 16 patients improved markedly or moderately. The spastic postural disorders of the lower limbs, like hyperadduction, internal rotation, equinism etc. has been reduced or abolished. On the other hand it must be stressed that similar disorders were only slightly improved in two patients, in whom the disorder was only evident during voluntary movement.

Postural hyperextension was also reduced or abolished by the operation. Thus 3 patients acquired the sitting position (impossible before operation)—and one was markedly improved. In these cases the operation also involved the twelvth dorsal root.

In all cases of tetraspasticity, slight or moderate improvement of the mobility of the upper limbs and especially of the hands, was observed. Also in 3 patients improvement of speech, and in 1 of mastication, was observed.

Table 2. *Results of 16 Bilateral Posterior Partial Root Section D_{12}-S_1 or L_1-S_1 (Rhizotomy)*

Condition	Type of spasticity	Markedly improved	Improved	Slightly improved	Worsened	Sensation
Infantile cerebral diplegia	phasic			1		Superficial: Normal in all patients except 5, in whom negligible areas of hypoesthesia in some dermatomerus occurred
	tonic	2	1			
	mixed		2	1		
Infantile cerebral quadriplegia	tonic	4			1	
	mixed		2			
Post-traumatic spastic paraplegia	mixed		1			Deep: Reduction of lower limbs sense position (ataxy) in 3 of the 7 patients who could be studied with certainty
Spastic-dystonic syndrome				1		
Totals		6	6	3	1	

In all cases deep reflexes were markedly reduced or, more often, abolished. In only two cases they reappeared pathologically. In one patient, after 3 months, clonus in one foot reappeared at the same time as the equinus deformity. In another after three months polyphasic reflexes of the adductors, hyperadduction and internal rotation of the lower limbs simultaneously reappeared.

Clinical examination after operation showed superficial sensation to be normal in all patients, except in 5, in whom areas of hypoaesthesia in some dermatomes were observed. This rapidly lessened after some weeks or months.

Because of intellectual difficulties of the majority of the patients deep sensation could be evaluated with certainty in only 7 patients. In 4 of them this appeared normal, while in 3 others a moderate hypopallesthesia and reduction of position sense in the limbs was observed.

One patient showed a transient increase of the lower-limb paresis together with retention of urine. These complications were resolved after removing meningeal adhesions which were impeding the cerebro-spinal fluid circulation.

The only general complications observed in this series was a transitory bronchopneumonia in one patient and an anxiety depression syndrome in another probably caused by undue optimism as to the outcome of the operation.

Posterior Partial Rootlet Section (Radiclotomy)

Between January 1973 and February 1975, 24 spastic patients were operated on using the method of Foerster [2], but modified by the authors [5], that is partial section of the rootlets that constitute the posterior roots close to the cord. Our technique is different from another one recently proposed [15], in which the rootlets are partially cut within the spinal cord.

In 6 patients, radiclotomy was performed from D_{12} to S_1, while in the other 18 from L_1 to S_1.

The patients' ages ranged from 6 to 16 years and in all, except one, the etiology of the spastic syndrome was concerned with the usual perinatal pathology.

The clinical picture was stable in all cases, and was concerned with infantile spastic diplegia in 10 patients, infantile spastic quadriplegia in 13 and with one patient suffering from post-traumatic spastic paraplegia.

In general the spastic syndromes of this group of patients were less serious than those of the previous one, and, in particular, two patients were able to walk unaided. Moreover all patients had a normal or slightly reduced mental development.

The functional results obtained in these patients are reported in Table 3. In all patients, except two, marked or moderate improvement occurred, that is the operation resulted in reduction or abolition of spastic postural disorders of the lower limbs (e.g., hyperadduction, internal rotation, equinus deformity, etc.). It must be stressed that the only two patients who did not improve after the operation, showed spastic disorders of the lower limbs which were evident only with voluntary movements.

As in the previous series, the operation was able to reduce or abolish hyperextension of the trunk and to improve (slightly or moderately) mobility of the upper limbs in the quadriplegic syndromes. In two patients of this series a moderate improvement of speech was also observed.

The deep reflexes were abolished or markedly reduced in all patients.

Exteroceptive sensation appeared normal in all patients, except one, in whom hypoaesthesia over the dorsum of the feet was found. This defect was no longer present after 3 months.

Table 3. *Results of 24 Bilateral Posterior Partial Rootlet Section D_{12}-S_1 or L_1-S_1 (Radiclotomy)*

Condition	Type of spasticity	Markedly improved	Improved	Slightly improved	Sensation
Infantile cerebral quadriplegia	phasic tonic mixed	4	4	1 1	Superficial: Normal in all patients
Infantile cerebral diplegia	tonic mixed	5 2	3 3		
Post-traumatic spastic paraplegia	mixed		1		Deep: Normal in all patients
Totals		11	11	2	

Deep sensation could be evaluated unequivally in 20 out of 24 patients and in all cases, except one, appeared normal. Only one patient showed a reduction of the sense of position of the lower limbs, which was no longer present after 3 months.

No general complications were observed in this series.

Posterior Cervical Rhizotomy

Between April 1973 and February 1975, 16 patients suffering from dystonic and dystonic-athetoid syndromes were operated on by complete bilateral section of the first posterior cervical roots, an operation already performed for the same syndromes by Kottke [12] and Heimburger *et al.* [11].

All patients were operated under general anaesthesia using endotracheal intubation: the first 7 of this series were operated on using assisted respiration, while the other 9 had spontaneous respiration.

In 7 patients a laminectomy from C_1 to C_3 was performed; in another seven from C_1 to C_4 and the other two from C_1 to C_5. After opening the dura mater, it was noticed that the posterior root C_1 was absent bilaterally in 6 patients, absent unilaterally in 4 others, while in 5 patients it was present bilaterally, in the form of a large single fascicle which was not divided into rootlets at the entrance to the spinal cord.

In 7 patients, all the rootlets which constituted the posterior roots C_1-C_2-C_3 and some of the posterior rootlets of C_4 were cut; in another 7 patients the rhizotomy was extended also to some of the posterior rootlets of C_5 and in the other two patients some of the rootlets of C_6 were also cut. In 4 patients the external branch of the XI cranial nerve was also cut unilaterally. In one other patient bilateral section of the first two motor roots was performed, in addition to posterior cervical rhizotomy.

Table 4. *Results of 16 Bilateral Posterior Cervical Rhizotomy*

Condition	Markedly improved	Improved	Slightly improved	Worsened	Complications	Dead
Dystonic-athetoid syndromes	1 *	3	1		1 Cheyne-Stokes resp. in the early 2 post-op. hours Bronchopneumonia	1 Broncho-pneumonia
Dystonic-athetoid spastic syndromes		3	1		1 Broncho-pneumonia 1 Cheyne-Stokes resp. in the early 3 post-op. hours	
Dystonia		3	2	1	1 Broncho-pneumonia Cheyne-Stokes resp. in the early 6 post-op. hours	
Totals	1	9	4	1	4	1

* Operated on before by stereotactic dentatolysis.

As shown in Table 4, 4 patients improved slightly after the operation, 9 improved moderately and one, operated on previously by stereotactic dentatolysis, improved markedly. Thus the majority of patients, some weeks after the operation, showed a better sitting posture, better control of the head and more coordinated mobility of the upper and lower limbs. In 2 patients an improvement of walking was evident.

From a neurological point of view, reduction of dystonia and athetosis was more or less the same. It should be noticed that there was a moderate improvement of the upper limb and trunk dystonia and a less evident improvement of lower-limb dystonia. It should be further noted that head-dystonia improved, more or less to the same degree, as the upper limb and trunk dystonia and that, even if it was prevalent on one side, it did not improve any more by cutting unilaterally the external branch of the XI cranial nerve, in addition to posterior cervical rhizotomy.

Table 5. *Results of 21 Stereotactic Pulvinolyses and 3 Associated Lesions of the Lateralis Posterior Nucleus on 13 Patients*

Syndrome	Markedly improved	Improved	Slightly improved or unchanged	Total
Dystonia	2 *	2		4
Choreoathetosis		2	3	5
Infantile spastic quadriplegia			4	4
	2	4	7	13

* Operated on before by stereotactic dentatolysis.

There was a worsening of symptoms in the only patient operated on by bilateral section of the first two motor roots in addition to posterior cervical rhizotomy. This patient showed an excessive reduction of tone in the neck muscles which resulted in an aggravation of the head position, permanently in marked hyperextension.

Among the other neurological complications, paraesthesias in the upper limbs were noticed in a patient in whom rhizotomy was extended to C_6. This same patient developed an anxiety depression syndrome, probably caused by overoptimism regarding the outcome of the operation.

Among the general complications, bronchopneumonia occurred in 3 patients, but was cured on average in two weeks. On the contrary one other patient died from this illness five days after the operation.

During recovery from anaesthesia Cheyne-Stokes respiration, with long pauses, occurred in 3 patients but ceased completely 2, 3, and 6 hours afterwards.

In conclusion, posterior cervical rhizotomy is a useful operation for the reduction of dystonia and athetosis. Its most serious complications are in postoperative respiratory disturbances, especially in patients with pre-existing respiratory insufficiency.

Stereotactic Pulvinolysis

From November 1972 to April 1973 we performed 21 stereotactic pulvinolyses on 13 dyskinetic patients (Table 5). The operation was unilateral in 5 patients and bilateral in 8. In all cases the lesions were concerned both with the lateral and medial parts of the pulvinar and in 3 cases also in association with the posterior-lateral nucleus.

Operations were performed under general anaesthesia on 13 patients and under local anaesthesia on 5. In all cases, pneumoencephalography by the lumbar route was carried out to visualize the 3rd ventricle.

According to the stereotactic coordinates of Cooper et al. [1], the target centre of the pulvinar on the lateral projections of the radiograms was placed at a point 17–19 mm behind the midpoint of the commissural line and 4 mm above. This usually coincides with a point situated 4 mm behind and 4 mm above the posterior commissure. The distance from the mid-line was taken at 12 and 16 mm for medial and lateral pulvinar lesions, respectively. The centre target of the postero-lateral nucleus was taken at 12 mm behind the midpoint of the commissural line and 10 mm above on the lateral projections of the radiograms, and the distance from the mid-line was 15 mm.

As shown in Table 5, in 2 patients suffering from dystonic syndromes, stereotactic pulvinolysis, bilaterally performed in both cases, yielded a moderate improvement of the clinical symptomatology, that is a more co-ordinated mobility of the limbs and better control of the head and trunk. In 2 other dystonic patients, operated on previously by bilateral stereotactic dentatolysis, the lesion of pulvinar, unilateral in 1 case and bilateral in the other, increased the improvement, and the final results were very satisfactory. In fact, both these patients, even if they could not stand alone (disturbance of equilibrium associated with the dyskinetic syndromes), acquired an independent sitting posture and could bring some food to the mouth.

In 5 patients suffering from choreoathetosis, bilateral stereotactic pulvinolysis in 3 and unilateral in 2 were performed. In 1 of 2 patients operated on unilaterally, a lesion of the postero-lateral nucleus was also performed. In this group of patients moderate improvements in two and slight in one were observed, of the 3 patients who showed a prevalence of choreic components; while no improvement was observed in the 2 patients who showed a prevalence of the athetoid component.

There was no obvious improvement in 4 patients suffering from infantile spastic quadriplegia, in 2 of whom pulvinolysis was bilateral and in 2 unilateral with an associated lesion of the postero-lateral nucleus.

Of the complications only one patient showed a postoperative hemiparesis, which partially improved in the following months.

A review of the operation showed that the lesion involved the internal capsule.

From our experience we do not believe that the pulvinar plays an important role in spasticity. In fact, not one of the spastic patients operated on by stereotactic pulvinolysis, whether or not there was a lesion of the postero-lateral nucleus, had noticeable improvement after the operation. Neither was there variation of muscular tone in those patients who were operated on by us using the same operation for intractable pain [6].

Table 6. *Results of 6 Unilateral Stereotactic Associated V. L. Thalamolysis and Pulvinolysis*

Condition	Markedly improved	Improved	Slightly improved
Unilateral dystonic-athetoid Syndromes		2	
Dystonia		1	1
Choreoathetosis		1	1
Totals		4	2

In our experience of the choreoathetotic syndromes the role of the pulvinar is questionable. We have observed some slight or moderate improvement in those syndromes in which the choreic component was prevalent. On the contrary, in dystonic syndromes stereotactic pulvinolysis yielded more favourable results but of moderate degree. However, we consider that for these syndromes, stereotactic dentatolysis is the preferred operation, both because of the more demonstrated role of the dentate nucleus and because of our own experience of better results.

However, one operation is often insufficient to obtain effective results it seems to us that stereotactic pulvinolysis can add to the benefits of stereotactic dentatolysis in dystonic syndromes.

Stereotactic Associated V.L. Thalamolysis and Pulvinolysis

In 1974, 6 patients suffering from dyskinetic syndromes which were more marked on one side (dystonic, dystonic-athetoid or choreoathetoid) were operated on with controlateral stereotactic lesions of the V.L. nucleus and pulvinar.

As shown in Table 6, in 4 patients there was a moderate reduction of athetosis and dystonia, with improved use of the limbs. While in the other two only slight improvement was observed.

Conclusion

One hundred and twenty-two patients suffering from spasticity and/or dyskinesias underwent one or more operation, among which there were 88 stereotactic dentatolyses, 24 posterior partial rootlet sections D_{12}-S_1 or L_1-S_1, 16 posterior partial root sections D_{12}-S_1 or L_1-S_1, 16 posterior cervical rhizotomies, 21 stereotactic pulvinolyses, 6 stereotactic associated V.L. thalamolyses and pulvinolyses.

Evaluating the results obtained from these operations, it can be seen that spastic syndromes of the "tonic" type improve with partial posterior rhizotomy. The same favourable results for "tonic" spasticity are obtained with partial posterior rootlet section, that is with a less aggressive technique. Because of the sparing of deep sensation this operation can be performed even in spastic patients who are acquiring or have already acquired independent standing or walking.

Among the stereotactic operations capable of reducing spasticity, we believe that only dentatolysis merits further study, but only for certain syndromes, such as infantile spastic hemiparesis or paraparesis of "phasic" or "mixed" type. While on the other hand we do not consider that the pulvinar plays an important role in spasticity.

Regarding dystonic and dystonic-athetoid syndromes, it should be noticed that, if only one operation is often insufficient to obtain good functional results, several operations are capable of reducing dystonia and athetosis. These operations, which can be associated in our experience are in order of effectiveness: bilateral stereotactic dentatolysis, posterior cervical rhizotomy, stereotactic pulvinolysis associated to V.L. thalamolysis.

References

1. Cooper, I. S., Amin, I., Chandra, R., Waltz, I. M. (1973), A surgical investigation of the clinical physiology of the L.P.-pulvinar complex in man. J. neurol. Sci. *18*, 89—110.
2. Foerster, O. (1908), Über eine neue operative Methode der Behandlung spastischer Lähmungen mittels Resektion hinterer R.M.-Wurzeln. Z. Orthop. Chir. *22*, 202—223.
3. Fraioli, B. (1973), Spasticità: problemi fisiopatologici, clinici e terapeutici. Riv. Neurol. *43*, 196—228.
4. Fraioli, B., Guidetti, B., La Torre, E. (1973), The stereotaxic dentatotomy in the treatment of spasticity and dyskinetic disorders. J. Neurosurg. Sci. *17*, 49—52.
5. Fraioli, B., Guidetti, B. (1975), La rizotomia posteriore parziale e una nuova tecnica, la radicolotomia posteriore parziale, nel trattamento della spasticità tonica. Riv. Pat. Nerv. Ment. *99*, 118—135.

6. Fraioli, B., Guidetti, B. (1975), Effects of stereotactic lesions of the pulvinar and lateralis posterior nucleus on intractable pain and dyskinetic syndromes of man. Appl. Neurophysiol. *38*, 23—30.
7. Gros, C., Ouaknine, G., Vlahovitch, B., Frerebeau, Ph. (1967), La radicotomie sélective postérieure dans le traitement neuro-chirurgical de l'hypertonie pyramidale. Neurochirurgie *13*, 505—518.
8. Guidetti, B., Moscatelli, G. (1963), Gli esami radiografici negli interventi stereotassici; note tecniche sull'uso di un apparecchio costruito per la realizzazione di esami di precisione. Lav. Neuropsichiat. *41*, 1—10.
9. Heimburger, R. F., Whitlock, C. C. (1965), Stereotaxic destruction of the human dentate nucleus. Confin. Neurol. (Basel) *26*, 346—358.
10. Heimburger, R. F. (1969), The role of the cerebellar nuclei in dyskinetic disorders. Confin. Neurol. (Basel) *31*, 57—72.
11. Heimburger, R. F., Slominski, A., Griswold, P. (1973), Posterior cervical rhizotomy for reducing spasticity in cerebral palsy. J. Neurosurg. *39*, 30—34.
12. Kottke, F. J. (1970), Modification of athetosis by denervation of the tonic neck reflexes. Develop. Med. Child. Neurol. *12*, 236—237.
13. Nashold, B. S., Slaughter, D. G. (1969), Effects of stimulating or destroying the deep cerebellar regions in man. J. Neurosurg. *31*, 172—186.
14. Siegfried, J., Esslen, E., Gretener, U., et al. (1970), Functional anatomy of the dentate nucleus in the light of stereotaxic operations. Confin. Neurol. (Basel) *32*, 1—10.
15. Sindou, M., Fischer, G., Goutelle, A., Schott, B., Mansuy, L. (1974), La radicellotomie postérieure sélective dans le traitement des spasticités. Rev. Neurol. *130*, 201—216.
16. Zervas, N. T., Horner, F. A., Pickren, K. S. (1967), The treatment of dyskinesia by stereotaxic dentatectomy. Confin. Neurol. (Basel) *29*, 93—100.

Author's address: Dr. B. Guidetti, Istituto di Neurochirurgia, Viale Università 30, I-00185 Rome, Italy.

Acta Neurochirurgica, Suppl. 24, 41—48 (1977)

Department of Neurological Surgery, Kantonsspital,
University of Zürich, Switzerland

Long-Term Assessment of Stereotactic Dentatotomy for Spasticity and Other Disorders

J. Siegfried and J. C. Verdie

With 2 Figures

Summary

In the 60's stereotactic electrocoagulation of the dentate nucleus became a promising approach in the neurosurgical treatment of muscular hypertonicity, particularly when spasticity was evident. A relatively satisfactory improvement of spasticity has been reported earlier as a result and the authors were supporting these clinical results in previous publications. A long-term assessment of the results obtained in a large series of patients would permit a better evaluation of the effect of the operation. Analysing 109 stereotactic electrocoagulations of the dentate nucleus on 50 patients mainly in cases of cerebral palsy over a period of more than 10 years (most patients underwent a bilateral dentatotomy), the authors give a more realistic appreciation of the results, which depend on the criteria chosen. In 30% of the cases a clear improvement in the spasticity was obtained, and in 50% of all cases, nursing and rehabilitation were facilitated. The stereotactic dentatotomy never completely cured the spasticity and spectacular results were never observed, but the operation can be performed without complications and an unexpected neurological deficit did not occur. The role of the stereotactic dentatotomy and other neurosurgical methods in the treatment of spasticity has to be evaluated more critically.

Introduction

The first attempt of selective destruction of the dentate nucleus was made by Delmas-Marsalet and van Bogaert [4] forty years ago. In a Parkinsonian patient, they destroyed the dentate nucleus by means of a hook introduced through a small burr hole. The unfortunate results, with myoclonic syndrome, nystagmus, severe swallowing troubles, hemiplegia on the right side with loss of sensation, aggravation of tremor and finally the death of patient on 9th postoperative day discouraged further new approaches of this nucleus for several years.

The first paper on results obtained by stereotactic dentatotomy (the first case being operated on 1963) was published by Heimburger [11]. This resulted in a renewal of interest in the stereotactic treatment of some functional disorders, particularly in those of spasticity from cerebral palsy. Between 1965 and 1969, there were many publications on this topic, but dentatotomy never became as

Table 1. *Clinical Syndromes Presented by the 50 Cases Operated on*

Athetosis double	13
Little's disease	8
Spasmodic tetraplegia	7
Dystonia	6
Choreoathetosis	4
Spasmodic hemiplegia	3
Hemi-athetosis	1
Disseminated sclerosis	2
Spasmodic torticollis	2
Ramsay-Hunt	1
Various (spasticity in case of diseases not labelled)	3
	50

popular as thalamotomy in cases of tremor. During the past 5 years, the interest in this technique declined markedly and the enthusiasm of 10 years ago practically disappeared and was replaced by scepticism. Since we had the opportunity during the past 8 years to operate on a rather large series of patients, it seemed appropriate to analyse with follow-up from 3 to 8 years the value of stereotactic dentatotomy for spasticity and other abnormal condition in 50 patients.

Material

50 patients (27 males and 23 females) operated on between May, 1967 and June, 1972 were selected, on the basis that the history was adequately documented. 42 cases of cerebral palsy with a spastic component represented the main indication for surgery. Table 1 gives the distribution of all the cases, but we know how difficult it is to put a precise diagnosis in case of cerebral palsy. The age of patients at the time of the operation is shown in Fig. 1. The first peak corresponds exclusively to cases of cerebral palsy.

Methods

All dentatotomies were performed stereotactically with Riechert's frame used upside down. A good visualization of the IVth ventricle is obtained at the time of operation by means of fractioned pneumoencephalography with the patients in sitting position. Stereotactic anatomy of the dentate nucleus is still controversial. As a target, we chose a point 10 mm behind the line tangent to the floor of the IVth ventricle, 5 mm below the line perpendicular to the floor of the IVth ventricle passing through the apex of this structure and 14 mm laterally to the midline. A directional burr hole (stereo-

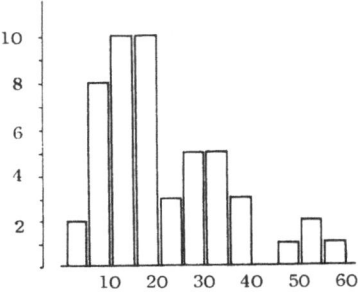

Fig. 1. Age of the 50 patients at the time of the operation

tactically) is made with a dental drill of 2 mm diameter and the electrode introduced at an appropriate angle to penetrate the dentate nucleus in the frontal and sagittal main axis. Three to six high frequency coagulations are then performed and the lesion could be extended with adjacent directionally oriented coagulations using a side electrode.

The operation was performed unilaterally only on 9 cases of hemisyndrome or in cases where symptoms were very marked on one side. In the beginning the bilateral dentatotomy was made in two sessions, but since 1969, it is performed in one stage. Reoperation was indicated in 9 cases. Therefore, a total of 109 dentate nucleus lesions were performed.

The clinical assessment of the results of stereotactic procedures for functional disorders is rather difficult, and the criteria chosen can be only analysed subjectively. We are using a rating scale which is summarized in Table 2. The rating scale was used before the operation, after 6 months (short follow-up), after 2 years (middle follow-up) and after at least 3 years up to 8 years (long follow-up). The 4 grades of the scale not only reflect the clinical symptoms but are also the translation of a function. The goal of this surgery is a functional one and the recovery of one function is more important than the aesthetic result.

Results

Five patients were by no means improved by the operation (Fig. 2 and Table 3): Two cases of spamodic torticollis, 2 cases of dystonia and one case of myoclonia (Ramsay Hunt). Thirty patients (60%) had a very good result 6 months after the operation, but 2 years later their number dropped to 16 (32%). Slight improvement but not satisfactory was noticed after 6 months in 15 cases (30%). Among them 4 lost the benefit from the operation after 2 years. However, after 2 years, 50% of the patients had a slight improvement, since we are including in this number the 14 cases who had a better

Table 2. *Rating Scale Used in the Evaluation of the Results*

Grade	Clinical observation
3	Suppression or very marked improvement of practically all symptoms, particularly the spasticity and the hyperkinesias. Very good functional result
2	Satisfactory functional result. Symptoms improved, but still pronounced
1	Slight improvement of symptom and function. Nursing and rehabilitation facilitated
0	No effect

result after 6 months but not long lasting. This slight improvement facilitated nursing care and rehabilitation. We know that amelioration of the symptomatology after stereotactic dentatotomy is more marked in the months immediately following the operation, but the follow-up study over the years shows that the rate of improvement is decreasing and this is particularly true in the cases which improved clearly after 6 months. If after 6 months we had 10% failures, after 2 years the failure rate reached 20% of the cases and after 3 years 24% (Fig. 2). No difference can be seen if the stereotactic dentatotomy is made in one or two sessions. Some patients underwent a stereotactic operation (pallidotomy, thalamotomy) before the dentatotomy. These cases are irrelevant since the evaluation of successes or failures are attributed directly to the dentatotomy. Five patients were operated later on for further improvement of functional disorders. In 3 cases, a ventrolateral thalamotomy did not change the spasticity component, if present, but had a favorable effect on the hyperkinesias. In one case, a pulvinarotomy combined with a ventrolateral thalamotomy helped to regain the decreasing improvement from dentatotomy with long lasting success.

Looking for the success in relation to the clinical picture (Table 3), the choreathetosis show surprisingly good results, but the number of cases are to small for critical judgment. The best surgical indication seems to be a syndrome with congenital spasticity (Little's disease and spasmodic tetra- or hemiplegia): about 50% of the cases had a fairly good result. Dystonia musculorum deformans seems to be a

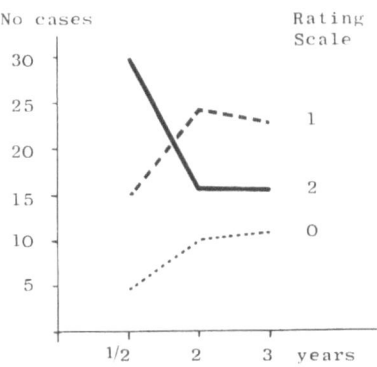

Fig. 2. Effect of dentatotomy on the rating scale of all 50 patients after 6 months, 2 years and 3 years

poor indication. This is also true for spasmodic torticollis and for spasticity of multiple sclerosis, but the number of cases operated on is small.

Two transitory complications has to be mentioned. In one case of Little's disease, postoperative nystagmus and intention tremor of the hands were observed for a few days. On re-checking the per-operative X-rays of these cases, we have the impression that the coagulation were to high and too medial. In other words, the lesion probably reached the medial nuclei (Nucleus globosus, nucleus emboli-formis and maybe nucleus fastigius). In a 4 years old child suffering from spastic tetraplegia, a bilateral dentatotomy resulted in a total disappearance of spasticity. Fortunately, few months later, some spastic components reappeared giving a fairly good functional result.

Discussion

Reports on long follow-up of large series of patients suffering from spasticity and involuntary movements and operated on with a dentatotomy are rare. The largest series is reported by Heim-burger [7, 8, 9, 10, 11]. In their last paper, the author reports the results observed in a series of 64 patients, with an overall moderate improvement in 46 cases. The group of spastic diplegia (Little's disease) and hemiplegia give the most impressive successes and we quite agree with this interpretation. However, it seems to us that the results which were satisfactory a few months after the operation are not as good 2 years or more later. In our previous papers we reported encouraging results [15, 16, 17, 18, 19, 20, 21, 22, 23]. Now our impression is

Table 3. *Clear Improvement (Long Lasting Grade 2 of the Rating Scale) According to the Clinical Picture*

	No of cases improved	In per cent of cases operated on
Little's disease, Spasmodic tetraplegia and hemiplegia	8	44%
Athetosis (hemi- or double)	4	28%
Choreoathetosis	3	75%
Dystonia	0	0%
Disseminated sclerosis	0	0%
Spasmodic torticollis	0	0%
Various	0	0%

that the long term follow-up is definitely not so satisfactory as the results few months after the operation. The others publications in the literature are so far mainly related to clinical results analysed a few months after the stereotactic dentatotomies and thus are quite comparable to our primary observations [1, 3, 5, 6, 12, 13, 14, 24, 25]. Reassessment revealed to us that long lasting successes from dentatotomy are very rare and never spectacular.

A definite correlation between symptomatology, age of patient and duration of the disease is not possible. The most important controls missing are the location of the coagulation within the dentate nucleus and the size of the lesion. We do not have a single control or postmortem examination in our whole series. A reconstruction of the radiological site of the coagulation would be worthwile and its correlation with the clinical result has still to be done. We still feel, that the best results were obtained with coagulations in the more ventrolateral part [22]. It is possible that practically many of our coagulations are too small and maybe not in the ideal part of the dentate nucleus. But we know that functionally, an improvement of the spasticity, even if only slight, is better than a complete disappearance of this symptom: a child with cerebral palsy can learn to walk with a spastic paraparesis, but not with an atonic one.

The place of stereotactic dentatotomy in the neurosurgical treatment of spasticity and of dyskinesias other than tremors is a limited one. For involuntary movements, a ventrolateral thalamotomy or a subthalamotomy give much better results. The only disadvantage of this last operation is the very frequent undesirable complications when used bilaterally and thus has to be done only unilaterally. However, dentatotomy may result in more improvement of the involuntary movements of the trunk. Dentatotomy provides the best success in alleviating spasticity. Its success must not be over rated; it is moderate and decreases over the years. But this method is safe, can be done bilaterally in one session and complications are very rare. Its place in the future of functional neurosurgery is questionable. New technics are, for the time being, more promising. The dorsal column stimulation for spasticity has already shown encouraging results [2] and our own experience in 3 cases (among them 2 cases of multiple sclerosis followed up only 8 and 6 months) have so far good results and this cannot be overlooked.

References

1. Balasubramaniam, V., Kanaka, T. S., Ramanujam, P. B. (1974), Stereotaxic surgery for cerebral palsy. J. Neurosurg. *40*, 577—582.
2. Cook, A. W., Weinstein, S. P. (1973), Chronic dorsal column stimulation in multiple sclerosis. New York State J. Med. *73*, 2868—2872.
3. D'Andrea, F., Ferrari, E., Divitis, E., Mattioli, G. (1966), Effeti immediati e tardivi della coagulazione stereotassica mono e bilaterale del nucleo dentato sulla „dissinergia cerebrale mioclonica". Min. Neurochir. *10*, 375—379.
4. Delmas-Marsalet, P., Bogaert, L. van (1935), Sur un cas de myoclonies rhythmiques continues déterminées par une intervention chirurgicale sur le tronc cérébral. Rev. Neurol. *64*, 728—740.
5. Divitis, E., Signorelli, L. D., Cerillo, A. (1972), Stereotaxic surgery for nonparkinsonian dyskinesias. Neurochirurgia *15*, 92—95.
6. Fraioli, B., Guidetti, B., La Torre, E. (1974), The stereotaxic dentatotomy in the treatment of spasticity and dyskinetic disorders. J. neurol. Sci. 49—52.
7. Heimburger, R. F. (1967), Dentatectomy in the treatment of dyskinetic disorders. Confin. Neurol. (Basel) *29*, 101—106.
8. Heimburger, R. F. (1969), The role of the cerebellar nuclei in dyskinetic disorders. Confin. Neurol. (Basel) *31*, 57—72.
9. Heimburger, R. F. (1970), The cerebellum and spasticity. Int. J. Neurol. *7*, 232—243.
10. Heimburger, R. F. (1970), The role of the cerebellar nuclei in spasticity. Confin. Neurol. (Basel) *32*, 105—113.
11. Heimburger, R. F., Whitlock, C. C. (1965), Stereotaxic destruction of the human dentate nucleus. Confin. Neurol. (Basel) *26*, 346—358.
12. Nádvorník, P., Šramka, M., Lisy, L., Svicka, I. (1972), Experiences with dentatotomy. Confin. Neurol. (Basel) *34*, 320—324.
13. Nádvorník, P., Šramka, M. (1973), Transtentorial dentatotomy in "Recent progress in neurological surgery". Excerpta Medica *293*, 19.
14. Nashold, B. S., Slaughter, D. G. (1969), Effects of stimulating and destroying the deep cerebellar regions in man. J. Neurosurg. *31*, 172—186.

15. Krayenbühl, H., Siegfried, J. (1969), La chirurgie stéréotaxique du noyau dentelé dans le traitement des hyperkinésies et des états spastiques. Neuro-Chirurgie *15*, 51—58.
16. Krayenbühl, H., Siegfried, J. (1972), Dentatotomies or thalamotomies in the treatment of hyperkinesia. Confin. Neurol. (Basel) *34*, 29—33.
17. Siegfried, J. (1970), L'apport de la neurochirurgie fonctionelle dans le traitement des infirmes moteurs cérébraux. Rev. Oto-Neuro-Ophtalm. *42*, 412—414.
18. Siegfried, J. (1971), Stereotaxic cerebellar surgery. Confin. Neurol. (Basel) *33*, 350—360.
19. Siegfried, J., Ketz, E., Trachtenberg, M. (1972), Stereotactic recording on the depth of the cerebellum. In: Neurophysiology studied in man (Somjen, ed.), Vol. 1, pp. 366—369. Amsterdam: Excerpta Medica.
20. Siegfried, J. (1972), Stereotactic treatment of hypertonicity. In: Present limits of neurosurgery (Fusek, I., Kunc, Z., eds.), Vol. 1, pp. 549—550. Prague: Avicenum.
21. Siegfried, J. (1974), Methods and results in spasticity and hyperkinesias. In: Recent progress in neurological surgery (Sano, K., Ishii, S., eds.), Vol. 1, pp. 251—255. Amsterdam: Excerpta Medica and New York: Elsevier.
22. Siegfried, J., Esslen, E., Gretener, U., Ketz, E., Perret, E. (1970), Functional anatomy of the dentate nucleus in the light of stereotaxic operations. Confin. Neurol. (Basel) *32*, 1—10.
23. Siegfried, J., Perret, E. (1968), La dentatotomie stéréotaxique: nouvelle méthode de traitement chirurgical des hyperkinésies. Rev. Oto-Neuro-Ophtalm. *40*, 341—343.
24. Zervas, N. T. (1970), Paramedial cerebellar nuclear lesions. Confin. Neurol. (Basel) *32*, 114—117.
25. Zervas, N. T., Horner, F. A., Pickren, K. S. (1967), The treatment of dyskinesias by stereotaxic dentatectomy. Confin. Neurol. (Basel) *29*, 93—100.

Author's address: Prof. Dr. J. Siegfried, Neurochirurgische Universitätsklinik, Kantonsspital, Rämistraße 100, CH-8091 Zürich, Switzerland.

Acta Neurochirurgica, Suppl. 24, 49—51 (1977)
© by Springer-Verlag 1977

Department of Neurosurgery, Beth Israel Hospital and Harvard Medical School,
Boston, U.S.A.

Long-Term Review of Dentatectomy in Dystonia Musculorum Deformans and Cerebral Palsy

N. T. Zervas

Since 1966 34 patients with disorders of movement and tone due to dystonia musculorum deformans, cerebral palsy and other dyskinesias underwent ablation of the cerebellar dentate nucleus. Long term results (2–8 years) in 19 patients could be verified. Five other patients died and 10 were lost to follow up. Table 1 lists the disease

Table 1. *Patient Classification*

Total number of patients	34
Cerebral palsy	20
Retrocollic cerebral palsy	3
Parkinsonism	3
Dystonia	4
Multiple sclerosis	1
Choreo-athetosis	3

classification of these patients. Unilateral dentate lesions were placed in all of these patients ipsilateral to the side of major symptomatology. The methodology employed was described in a previous communication [1].

Results

One patient died of respiratory insufficiency one month following operation. This patient had severe retrocollis due to cerebral palsy and had pre-existing severe pulmonary insufficiency. He was not benefited by operation and succumbed to bronchopneumonia. The cerebellar complications of the operation are described in Table 2. All subsided except in one patient, who had persistent ataxia following dentate ablation. This probably resulted from extension of the lesion into the vestibular nuclei, since some nystagmus was present as well. No patient developed late cerebellar ataxia.

Three patients underwent dentatectomy for parkinsonian rigidity and tremor. One patient was available for follow-up eight years following operation and continued to have relief of parkinsonian rigidity. However, the interpretation was clouded by the fact that the patient was also receiving Levodopa therapy.

Table 2. *Adverse Cerebellar Effects (34 Patients)*

	Immediate complications	Complications still present 2–8 years later
Hypotonia	3	0 (2)
Dysmetria	2	0 (2)
Ataxia (trunkal)	2	0 (2)
Ataxia (limb)	2	1 (2)

Key for Table 2: ( ) patients available for follow-up.

Four patients with dystonia musculorum deformans were operated upon. All had had prior thalamotomy. One had been lost to follow up and three were contacted. Table 3 describes the results over a two to eight year period in these latter patients and indicates that useful improvement in daily functions as well as dyskinesia was still apparent.

Table 3. *Dystonia*

	Early improved	Late examined	Late improved
Dyskinesia	3 (4)	3	2
Hypertonia	3 (4)	3	2
Feeding	2 (4)	3	1
Dressing	3 (4)	3	1
Ambulation	2 (4)	3	2

The patients with multiple sclerosis, choreo-athetosis and dystonic cerebral palsy with retrocollis were not benefited in either the short or long term.

The results were far less encouraging in 20 patients with cerebral palsy. Table 4 describes the early and long term results. It can be seen, that few if any of the patients developed any functional improvement although there was some discernible change in dyskinesia. All of these patients had severe incapacitating cerebral palsy and most were bedridden. Specifically, ambulation, dressing and feeding were scarcely improved in any patients either in the short or long term.

In summing up, it is clear that dentatectomy can help dyskinesia. This is shown in the experience with parkinsonian and dystonia patients. With such a limited series, however, it is difficult to predict with certainity the outcome of any patient, although symptoms such

Table 4. *Cerebral Palsy*

	Early improved	Late examined	Late improved
Dyskinesia	9 (16)	6	3
Hypertonia	3 (9)	2	0
Feeding	1 (20)	—	—
Dressing	1 (20)	—	—
Ambulation	0 (20)	—	—

Key for Tables 3 and 4: ( ) present prior to operation.

as retrocollis and axial deformity did not appear to respond at all to ablation of this nucleus.

I believe that thalamotomy is the initial procedure for most cases of dystonia musculorum deformans and that dentatectomy should be reserved as an adjunct for severe painful limb and axial posturing as a last resort. I do not believe that our results warrant further use of this procedure in patients with advanced cerebral palsy. Although it is true that motor performance can be altered to the initial enthusiasm of the family and nursing personnel, it is also clear that an objective verification of useful gains or reduced problems in management could not be made.

References

Zervas, N. T., Horner, F. A., Pickren, K. S. (1967), The treatment of dyskinesias by stereotaxic dentatectomy. Confin. Neurol. (Basel) *29*, 93—100.

Author's address: N. T. Zervas, M.D., Department of Neurosurgery, Beth Israel Hospital and Harvard Medical School, 330 Brookline Avenue, Boston, MA 02215, U.S.A.

Acta Neurochirurgica, Suppl. 24, 53—57 (1977)
© by Springer-Verlag 1977

Istituto di Neurochirurgia della Università di Torino, Italy

New Aspects in the Surgical Treatment of Cerebral Palsy

V. A. Fasano, R. Urciuoli, G. Broggi, G. Barolat-Romana, F. Benech, A. Ivaldi, and A. Sguazzi

Posterior Functional Rhizotomy

180 cases of cerebral palsy with spasticity have been surgically treated since 1971. Different surgical procedures were employed: Cryopulvinarectomy (22 cases), bilateral cryodentatolysis (48 cases), associated cryopulvinarectomy and bilateral cryodentatolysis (10 cases), Foerster's posterior rhizotomy (14 cases), selective posterior rhizotomy (24 cases), and functional posterior rhizotomy (62 cases).

Our experience shows that posterior lumbar rhizotomy is the most effective treatment of spasticity.

Selective posterior rhizotomy, as was suggested by Foerster, is actually a quantitatively partial rhizotomy, mostly saving dermatome innervation, while functional posterior rhizotomy consists in the selective interruption of pathological diffusion depending on the inability of the centers to deal with spinal circuits.

Functional posterior rhizotomy is done in a Faraday cage, with the aid of the intraoperative microscope. The basis of functional lumbar rhizotomy is the anatomical identification of each root and careful isolation of each rootlet at its entrance to the spinal cord.

Electrostimulation of the posterior lumbar roots was carried out, initially during operations for disc herniation in five patients. We employed stimulation frequencies from 1 to 50 stimulations/second. The voltage varied from 0.2 to 2 volts. With both 1 and 50 stimulations/second, the response was clinically characterized by a single muscular contraction, without diffusion. This was confirmed by EMG recordings.

In spastic patients responses were not uniform. We observed three types:

1. A single muscular contraction to both 1 and 50 stimulations/second.

2. A continuous tonic muscular contraction lasting the whole stimulation time. The EMG recording shows that every single stimulus of a dorsal root is followed by a single muscular contraction. This type of response has been observed mainly in patients with spasticity in extension.

3. A continuous muscular contraction with a lower limb triple flexion pattern, often associated with an "after discharge" phenomenon and diffusion to homo/controlateral and upper limbs muscle groups. These cases usually show a clinical picture of spasticity in flexion. The last two responses are considered to be pathological. Only the roots/rootlets showing such responses are sectioned.

As an example we report a case in which L 4 stimulation is followed by a mixed response, a single response of the quastrochemius followed by a diffuse lower limb triple flexion. The L 4 rootlet giving rise to the pathological triple flexion response is then searched for, and, when it is found, it is sectioned. L 4 stimulation is now followed by a single contraction of the gastronemius. After section there has been also an immediate fall in muscle tone. The stretch reflex is greatly reduced, too.

A detailed examination of the spinal circuits and a quantitative analysis of the pathological diffusion can be carried out by dividing the corresponding anterior and posterior roots. An analysis of the afferent pathway, by peripheral nerve stimulation, simultaneously recording from posterior and anterior roots, and the efferent pathway, recording on the anterior root and the responding muscle groups, can therefore be performed. In this way, the spinal circuit can also be examined, by dorsal root stimulation and recording from the anterior roots. In the case shown here, recording from five anterior lumbar roots follows peroneal nerve electrostimulation. The recording shows a different diffusion of the stimulus in the various roots. In L 2 and L 4 there is partial diffusion. In L 3 and L 5 a complete diffusion. The modifications observed can be considered as an mability of the upper centres to deal with the spinal circuits. Their intraoperative investigation can lead to a better physiopathological understanding and to a more defined therapeutic approach.

After functional posterior rhizotomy there are several effects on muscle tone:

1. A noticeable reduction of lower limbs hypertonia, without subsequent hypotonia.

2. Reduction of the tone of the upper limbs mainly affecting distal segments, with evident improvement in skilfull movement and coordination.

3. A correction of the anomalous distribution of trunk and neck muscle tone.

An improvement has also been noticed in mechanisms of phonation.

These results are permanent. It has been suggested that recurrences following Foerster's operation can be explained by the sparing of certain roots, so that new neuronal connections, by sprouting, can be produced. Because functional posterior rhizotomy selects these pathological circuits and interrupts them selectively, recurrences are therefore avoided. Postoperative rehabilitation, by activating a normal proprioceptive adjustment, should avoid further pathological sprouting.

The main difference between Foerster's rhizotomy and functional rhizotomy, is that, while in the former locomotory ataxia is a common complication, in the latter it has never been observed. This is due to the greater preservation of proprioceptive afferents.

The number of roots and rootlets sectioned in functional rhizotomy operations, as compared to selective rhizotomy, is very low. This means, on the one hand, a considerable saving of proprioceptive afferents necessary for maintaining correct postural and coordination control, and for keeping an anatomical pathway for motor rehabilitation. On the other hand, the great variability in the number of the sectioned roots, varying from case to case, indicates that the different types of diffusion observed after electrostimulation, are not strictly related to the roots, but rather to the kind of spasticity present in each single case.

The main indication for functional rhizotomy is Little's spastic paraparesis and the mixed forms in which spasticity is predominant. As the functional results extend to the upper limbs, the operation is indicated also in spastic tetraparesis. Dystonic forms, both postural and hyperkinetic, are not influenced. Hypotonic forms, with dynamic spasticity, constitute a formal contraindication for posterior rhizotomy.

In suitable cases, spasticity disappears immediately after the section of the roots. As intensive and long lasting physiotherapy is mandatory for consequent functional improvement and patients must be able to cooperate. The mental status of the patient is therefore exceedingly important for 9,000 functional results.

In our series, recurrence of spastecity has occurred in about 5%% of the cases. These occurred mainly in mixed forms, in which spasticity was associated with dystonia, and by hypotonic forms with dynamic spasticity.

Chronic Neuroelectrostimulation
of the Anterior Cerebellar Lobe

A 12 years old boy, mentally normal, lying in a supine position showed rigidity and a lack of coordination with slow limb movements. The basic clinical pattern appeared when standing. The head, neck and limbs became hypotonic; every movement a diffuse useless muscular contraction. The main physiopathological disturbance is not spasticity, nor a motor weakness, but rather a loss of the proprioceptive scheme. For this reason a voluntary movement did not link up with an adequate corresponding postural organization. The boy could not walk, even held up. Extension rigidity and an evident ataxia was present. Clinically this case can be classified as an hypotonic tetraplegia with motor and postural extension rigidity. The patient was surgically treated with chronic electrostimulation of the anterior cerebellar lobe. This operation was done on the neurophysiological data from Sherrington and Moruzzi, demonstrating an inhibition of extension decerebrate rigidity after its stimulation.

The operative technique consists in the implantation on the surface of the anterior lobe of the cerebellum 6 electrodes in a Dacron mesh. The electrodes are subcutaneously connected by two cables to a miniaturized radio-receiver inserted in a pocket on the right side of the thoracic cage. X-ray films show the electrodes, cables and the side of the implant of the radio-receiver. An external battery powered transmitter generates pulsed radio-frequency signals. These signals are led alternatively to two small loop antennae through flexible lead wires. The antennae are taped directly over the subcutaneous implanted radio-receiver. The receiver modulates the signals and delivers the stimulating pulses to the electrodes implanted on the cerebellum.

An EMG before and during stimulation shows a considerable reduction of the stretch reflex. An EEG immediately and two hours after stimulation shows a lowering of voltage of cortical activity and a disappearance of the spikes, associated with stimulation. As an immediate result, the boy gained a proprioceptive concept which allowed him to achieve a postural and standing reaction. The control of head and neck postural fixation was obtained. He was able to stand up without support on both sides, and started to move a few steps, though without coordination.

Three months after we had a further improvement, especially in movement and motor coordination. The boy has begun to walk with crutches, and he can easily set up his kinetic reaction and stand up leaning on one hand.

This method needs further confirmation from either the neurophysiological investigation or from the analysis of the results of further operations.

References

Bucy (1949), The precentral motor cortex. Urbana University of Illinois.

Fasano, Barolat-Romana, Ivaldi, Sguazzi (1976), La radicotomie postérieure fonctionelle dans le traitment de la spasticité cérébrale. Neurochirurgie 22, 23—34.

Freeman, Heimburger (1948), The surgical relief of spasticity in paraplegic patients. Peripheral nerve section, posterior rhizotomy and other procedures. J. Neurosurg. 5, 556—561.

Foerster (1908), Über eine neue operative Methode der Behandlung spastischer Lähmungen durch Resektion hinterer Rückenmarkwurzeln. Z. orthop. Chir., 203—223.

Gros, Frerebeau, Kuhner, Perez (1973), Technical modification in the Foerster's operation selective posterior lumbar roots section: the result of 18 years of practice. Montpellier. Communication at the International Congress of Neurological Surgery, Tokyo.

MacLadery, Teasdall, Park, Languth (1952), Electrophysiological studies of reflex activity in patients with lesions of the nervous system. I. Comparison of spinal motoneurone excitability following afferent nerve volley in normal persons and patients with upper motor neurone lesions. Bull. Hopkins Hospital 219—249.

Maimros (1962), Neurosurgical possibilities in the treatment of spasticity. Acta Neurol. Scand., Suppl. 3, 38, 103—109.

Ouaknine (1965), La Radicotomie Sélective Postérieure dans le traitement de l'hypertoni pyramidale. Travail de la Clinique Neuro-Chirurgicale, CHU Montpellier.

Pedersen (1969), Spasticity. American Lectures Series, n. 752.

Penzholz (1956), Chirurgische Eingriffe am Nervensystem bei spastischen Lähmungen. Zbl. Neurochir. 16, 331—342.

Pollock, Davies (1930), Reflex activities of decerebrate animal. J. Comp. Neurol. 50, 377—411.

Price, Hull, Buchwald (1971), Intracellular response of dorsal horn cells to cutaneous and sural A and C fiber stimuli. Exp. Neurol. 33, 291—309.

Ranson (1915), Conduction within the spinal cord of the afferent impulses producing pain and vasomotor reflexes. Amer. J. Physiol. 38, 121—152.

Sherrington (1898), Decerebrate rigidity and reflexes coordination of movement. J. Physiol. 22, 319—322.

Sindou, Fisher, Goutelle, Mansuy, Shott (1974), La radicellotomie postérieure dans le traitement des spasticités. Rev. Neurol. 130.

Spivy, Metcalf (1959), Differential effect of medial and lateral dorsal root sections upon subcortical evoked potentials. J. Neurophysiol. 22.

Tardieu (1964), Les feuillets de l'infirmité motrice cérébrale. As. Nationale des Infirmes Moteurs-cérébraux, Paris.

Vlahovitch, Fuentes (1975), Résultats de la radicellotomie sélective postérieure à l'ótage lombaire et cervical. Neurochir. 21.

Authors' address: Prof. V. A. Fasano, Istituto di Neurochirurgia della Università di Torino, Via Cherasco, 15, I-10126 Torino, Italy.

Acta Neurochirurgica, Suppl. 24, 59—63 (1977)
© by Springer-Verlag 1977

Department of Neurosurgery, Rigshospitalet, Copenhagen, Denmark

Chronic Cerebellar Stimulation in Spastic Choreo-Athetosis*

K. Vaernet

Cerebellar modification of hypertonus was first demonstrated in 1897, when Loewenthal and Horsley [9] and Sherrington [12] independently reported that decerebrate rigidity could be relaxed by stimulation of the anterior lobe of the cerebellum.

An important observation on this subject was made in 1950, when Moruzzi [10] established that the result of cerebellar stimulation was depending upon the frequency of the stimulation. Stimulation with frequencies of 10 cycles per second (cps) would increase the decerebrate rigidity, while stimulation with frequencies of 100 to 300 cps produced a decrease of hypertonus. He further found that repetitive stimuli were always necessary in order to elicit a change in tonus, so that the effect was probably dependent upon a temporal summation in reticular and spinal internuncial neurones.

A modulating effect of the cerebellum upon the motor functions of the cerebral cortex has also been demonstrated. Soriano and Fulton [13] in 1947 found that spasticity after ablation of cortical areas 4 and 6 is augmented by ablation also of the anterior lobe of the cerebellum.

The effect of cerebellar stimulation upon the cortical systems is also dependent upon the frequency of stimulation. Nulsen, Black, and Drake [11] found in the monkey that slow frequency stimulation of the cerebellum would inhibit cerebral motor activity, while fast frequency stimulation would facilitate such activity.

These effects are mediated via extensive cerebellar projections to widespread areas of cerebral cortex, as demonstrated by Henneman, Cooke, and Snider [7]. The projections are mainly from cerebellar lateral and posterior cortical areas to dentate nuclei, which through

* This project was supported by grants from "Krista og Viggo Petersens Fond" and "Frantz Hoffmanns Mindelegat".

the brachium conjunctivum project to the ventro-lateral thalamic nuclei and from these primarily to areas 4 and 6. Vermal and anterior cerebellar areas project mainly via fastigial, globose and emboliform nuclei to vestibular and medial reticular formation nuclei, and to interlaminar thalamic nuclei [1].

The mechanisms involved in the modifications of central nervous system activity, induced by cerebellar stimulation are as yet mainly unresolved. Eccles, Ito, and Szentagothai [4] have, however, demonstrated that stimulation of cerebellar cortex induced Purkinje cell discharge. Ito, Yoshida, and Obata [8] have demonstrated that the synaptic effect of Purkinje cell discharge is uniformly inhibitory. The axons of the Purkinje cells project primarily to the intra-cerebellar nuclei. According to Eccles et al. [4] the nucleofugal impulses of these intra-cerebellar nuclei (dentatus, fastigium, interpositus) are purely exitatory. It is thus conceivable that the effect of the activity of the Purkinje cells elicited by cerebellar cortical stimulation, is an inhibition of the intra-cerebellar nuclei.

Even if the exact mechanisms involved are not known, we can at present accept the experimental evidence in favour of the existence of a frequency modulation in the cerebellar cortex. And this evidence is supported by the preliminary clinical experiences with the effect of cerebellar stimulation in patients with choreo-athetosis.

The clinical application of chronic cerebellar stimulation began when Cooper [2] in New York in November 1972 implanted the first cerebellar stimulating electrodes in a patient with congenital choreo-athetosis. A definitive improvement in both hypertonia and voluntary motor function was noted in this patient after a few weeks of stimulation. In 1973 Cooper [5] reported that 12 of 15 patients with hypertonia due to cerebral palsy or stroke had significant improvement after cerebellar stimulation with a frequency of 200 cycles per second.

We have during the last year implanted the Cooper-Avery cerebellar stimulating system in 4 patients with congenital spastic choreo-athetosis.

The electrode array currently in use consists of a plate of silicone coated mesh with 4 pairs of platinum disc electrodes. Through a small suboccipital craniectomy, one of these arrays is applied to the superior surface of each anterior lobe of the cerebellum beneath the tentorium. The electrode arrays are by subcutaneous tunnelling each connected to a miniature radio reciever, placed in subcutaneous pockets just below each clavicle. The recievers are activated by trans-epidermal inductive coupling from transmitting loop antennas taped to the skin, directly over each reciever. The antennas are plugged into the transmitter which is generating a pulse-modified radio signal at a carrier frequency of 2.1 MHz. A special timing mechanism within the transmitter causes this signal first to feed one antenna for a number of minutes, and then the other for the same period. Consequently the cerebellum is stimulated continuously, but in two separate areas alternately.

On the basis of experience thus far it appears that a stimulus frequency of approximately 200 cycles per second is effective in reducing spasticity. The stimulation pulses delivered by the transmitter are rectangular, of one millisecond width. The output to each antenna is at present adjusted to 10 volts. The timing mechanism will alternate the signal between the antennas at 16 minutes interval.

The case histories of the four patients operated so far will be summarized.

Case No. 1 (V.K.R.): 16 years old female with congenital spastic choreo-athetosis, who is totally dependant, unable to speak. Undoubtedly somewhat mentally retarded, but able to spell and count by pointing with a stick held between her teeth. Severe hypertonia of the extremities and the body with frequent episodes of ophistotonus and continuous athetotic movements of all four extremities.

A cerebellar stimulating system was implanted in April 1974. For the next to two months there was a definite improvement of the hypertonia and the hyperkinesia. In June 1974 she was readmitted to the department of neurosurgery with fever, vomiting and papiloedema. A ventriculography revealed a subdural abcess over one of the cerebellar electrode arrays. The electrodes and the recievers were removed, and her condition has again regressed to the preoperative status.

Case No. 2 (P.N.): A 12 years old boy with congenital choreo-athetosis, who could just stand unsupported, but could not walk. Could just manage to eat sandwiches without help. He had only slight hypertonia. His hyperkinesias were more pronounced in the arms than in the legs, and were mainly of a choreatic type. He is intellectually within normal range. Cerebellar stimulating system implanted in June 1974. On follow up in January 1975 his choreiform movements were apparently fairly unchanged, but his voluntary movements and his coordination were considerably improved. He could now handle small objects and assemble various small parts in his toys. He could write legibly in block letters, which he had previously been quite unable to do. He complained that "my hands get so silly again", when he on occasion had to be without stimulation, e.g., because of antenna break-down. He could stand better, and had on occasion been able to walk a few steps without support. On the whole his arms, however, were much more improved than his legs. On the next follow up in june his progress seemet to have remained at the same level, without further improvement.

Case No. 3 (H.E.): 9 years old boy with congenital spastic choreo-athetosis. Moderately psychically retarded. Severe dysarthria with hardly intelligible speach. Severe universal fluctuating hypertonia with continuous choreo-athetotic movements of all extremities. Could not sit alone and only hold his head momentarily. A leftsided electrocoagulation of his ventrolateral thalamic nucleus and the pulvinar thalami was made in december 1972 with a temporary improvement of the function of his right arm, and according to his parents with a permanent improvement of his voice and his swallowing. Cerebellar stimulating system implanted november 1974. At follow up in may 1975 he was considerably improved. He had been sitting alone and unsupported in his parents car on the way to the hospital, a drive of several hours. Can now sit on a horse with only slight support on one leg, while he previously had to be supported by an arm around his waist. He is able to hold his head considerably better. There is a marked improvement of hypertonia and athetosis in the legs, a more moderate improvement of the upper extremities, but he is now able to guide his hands and grasp firm objects. He also speaks better and psychically he is more alert, responsive and even-tempered.

Case No. 4 (S.K.J.): 22 years old male with congenital spastic choreo-athetosis, who is moderately psychically retarded, but with a fairly good vocabulary and intelligible speach. Severe hypertonia and choreo-athetosis of all four extremities, some tendency to ophistotonus. Can manoeuvre his weel-chair fairly well. In February 1970 a right-sided electrocoagulation of the dentate nucleus was made, with marked temporary decrease of hypertonia in his right arm. In 1971 left-sided electrocoagulation of ventro-lateral thalamic nucleus without significant change in his condition.

A cerebellar stimulator was implanted in February 1975. On follow up in july 1975 he had less hypertonia and better control of voluntary movements of the upper extremities. There was no definite change in his lower extremities. The stimulation had, however, been rather irregularly applied, as he often would close the transmitter, which interfered with his walkie-talkie, which was his great hobby.

There has in all the patients been an unquestionable effect both on hypertonus and on voluntary motor function following the cerebellar stimulation. The effect seems, as also reported by Cooper et al. [3], to be increasing, at least over several months. As also reported by the same authors, it may take some weeks after the stimulation has been instituted before the effect becomes manifest. The effect has not been quite consistent in all the patients. It would appear that an apparently identical placement of the electrodes on the surface of the cerebellum, has resulted in a more pronounced effect upon the upper extremities in patients number 2 and 4, and upon the lower extremities in patient number 3. Cooper et al. [3] have reported similar observations in some of their patients.

Whether the present placement of the electrode arrays or the parameters of stimulation are optimal is of course not yet known. We also, as yet, have insufficient knowledge of the long term effect of the stimulation upon the neuronal elements of the cerebellum. Gilman et al. [6] have recently reported that they found severe neuronal damage in the cerebellar cortex of a monkey, which had recieved cerebellar stimulation, using approximately the same stimulation parameters as those employed in the patients. The stimulation was, however, in the monkey applied continuously through one pair of electrodes for seven hours per day during three months. Even if this stimulation schedule is considerably different from that used in the patients, these findings must of course be given serious consideration, and long term studies are being conducted with this purpose in Dr. Gilman's laboratory. Cooper et al. [3] have however in their series of patients, who have been stimulated for more than one year, not seen any undesirable motor, sensory or intellectual changes. And in one patient, who died of his primary disease after more than one year of stimulation, Cooper [2] did not find any significant neuronal damage in the cerebellum, which could be ascribed to the stimulation.

As there are in Coopers patients, no evident clinical signs of cerebellar damage, even after prolonged periods of stimulation, we do find it permissable to implant cerebellar stimulators in small series of severely handicapped patients, as the apparently best means at our disposal to relieve some of their disability.

References

1. Carpenter, M. B. (1972), Core text of neuranatomy. Baltimore: Williams & Wilkins Co.
2. Cooper, I. S. (1973), Personal communication.
3. Cooper, I. S., Amin, I., Gilman, S., Waltz, J. M. (1974), The effect of chronic stimulation of cerebellar cortex on epilepsy in man. In: The cerebellum, epilepsy and behaviour (Cooper, I. S., Riklan, Snider, eds.). New York: Plenum Press.
4. Eccles, J. C., Ito, M., Szentagothai, J. (1967), The cerebellum as a neuronal machine. New York: Springer Verlag Inc.
5. Editorial (1973), Cerebellar stimulation aids victims of intractable hypertonia and epilepsy. J.A.M.A. 225, 1441—1449.
6. Gilman, S., Dauth, G. W., Tennyson, V. M., Kremzner, L. T., Chronic cerebellar stimulation in the monkey. Preliminary Observations. In press.
7. Henneman, E., Cooke, P. M., Snider, R. S. (1953), Cerebellar projections to the cerebral cortex. Res. Publ. Ass. Nerv. Ment. Dis. 30, 317—333.
8. Ito, M., Yoshida, M., Obata, K. (1964), Monosynaptic inhibition of the intracerebellar nuclei induced from the cerebellar cortex. Experientia (Basel) 20, 575—576.
9. Loewenthal, M., Horsley, V. (1897), On the relation between the cerebellar and other centers. Proc. Roy. Soc. 61, 20—25.
10. Moruzzi, G. (1950), Problems in cerebellar physiology. Springfield, Ill.: Ch. C Thomas.
11. Nulsen, F., Black, S., Drake, C. (1948), Inhibition and facilitation of motor activity by the anterior cerebellum. Fed. Proc. 7, 86—87.
12. Sherrington, C. S. (1897), Double (antidrome) conduction in the central nervous system. Proc. Roy. Soc. 61, 243—146.
13. Soriano, V., Fulton, J. F. (1947), Interrelation between anterior lobe of the cerebellum and the motor area. Fed. Proc. 6, 207—208.

Author's address: K. Vaernet, M.D., Department of Neurosurgery, Rigshospitalet, Copenhagen, Denmark.

Acta Neurochirurgica, Suppl. 24, 65—66 (1977)

Division of Neurosurgery, University of Texas Medical School, Houston, Texas

Treatment of Spasmodic Torticollis
With Dorsal Column Stimulation

Ph. L. Gildenberg

Because of the consideration that spasmodic torticollis might be an aberration of tonic muscle reflexes, an attempt was made to alter the afferent input of the reflexes by high frequency stimulation of the dorsal part of the spinal cord at the C-2 level in patients with spasmodic torticollis.

In order to evaluate each individual patient, first a trial of transcutaneous or skin stimulation is applied to the neck. Then a flexible subarachnoid dorsal column stimulating electrode is inserted percutaneously from the lateral approach at the C-1,2 level so that it lies behind the upper cervical spinal cord. It can be left in place for as long as one or two weeks, and the patient can be walking about while trial stimulation is being performed.

If the patient responds to this type of stimulation and if the patient tolerates the use of the stimulating apparatus, a permanent dorsal column stimulating electrode can be surgically implanted at the C-1 level.

To date, eighteen patients with spasmodic torticollis have been evaluated for treatment with stimulation.

Two of the 18 patients responded satisfactorily enough to the transcutaneous stimulation so that they were treated by this means alone.

Ten patients were rejected from consideration of any type of stimulation because they either did not tolerate the stimulation, demonstrated sufficient psychological instability during the trial period so that they were considered to be poor risks, or did not respond with clinical improvement to the stimulation.

Thus, six patients who were evaluated with transcutaneous and then percutaneous dorsal column stimulation had permanent surgically implanted dorsal column stimulators for treatment of their spasmodic torticollis.

Of the 6 patients who were implanted, 4 have had quite satisfactory relief for a follow-up varying between 1 year and 2¹/₂ years. Interestingly, the patients subjectively feel better even if the head is not returned quite to the normal position and are less distressed by pulling sensations of the neck or painful muscle spasms.

One patient had what may well actually be dystonia musculorum deformans. Although there was a tonic rotation and extreme extension of the neck, there was also tilting and extension of the upper thorax and shoulders. At the time of her admission, she was completely disabled and bedridden, requiring complete nursing care and feeding. During the 7 month follow-up period, she was able to walk with a walker with great difficulty, but was able to feed herself and provide herself with some self care.

The sixth patient in the series had only very transient relief. A revision of the dorsal column stimulator was performed with no improvement and eventually his stimulator was removed. This patient remains completely disabled from his spasmodic torticollis.

In summary, a new method of treating spasmodic torticollis with transcutaneous stimulation or the implantation of a dorsal column stimulator has been described. Of 18 patients evaluated for use of stimulation, 2 were treated with transcutaneous stimulation and 6 had surgically implanted dorsal column stimulators. One patient has had an excellent result, three have had good results and one has had a poor result. An additional patient with dystonia musculorum deformans is far less disabled with the use of dorsal column stimulation.

Author's address: Ph. L. Gildenberg, M.D., Ph.D., Professor and Chief, Division of Neurosurgery, University of Texas Medical School, Houston, TX 77025, U.S.A.

Acta Neurochirurgica, Suppl. 24, 67—71 (1977)
© by Springer-Verlag 1977

Department of Neurosurgery, Centro de Traumatologia y Rehabilitación
de la Seguridad Social, Zaragoza, Spain

Percutaneous Rhizotomy of the Articular Nerve of Luschka for Low Back and Sciatic Pain

G. Flórez, J. Eiras, and S. Ucar

Summary

The results of percutaneous facet rhizotomy for the treatment of low back
and sciatic pain in 30 patients are reported. Satisfactory results were obtained in
76% of cases. No complications were found. This procedure should be tried in
every patient with low back and extremity pain and no major neurological deficit
before resorting to laminectomy.

Introduction

Prior to 1934 it was thought that most of the lumbosciatic syndromes resulted from disorders of either the spinal facets or of the sacroiliac joints [4, 7]. This way of thinking changed following Mixter and Barr's report of the "ruptured" disc syndrome and from then on most neurosurgeons and orthopedic surgeons believed that low back and sciatic pain resulted from "ruptured" disc or from a psychosomatic disorder.

Many structures can contribute to pain in the spine: periostium, ligaments, muscles, joints, nerve roots and branches of nerve roots to the first four entities [11]. Therefore, a "ruptured" disc is only a possible cause of pain. On the other hand, most of the patients with low back and sciatic pain do not have a truly "ruptured" disc but a degenerated disc which may be "bulging". They may have limitation of straight leg raising but not a major neurological deficit. Contrast studies usually show a small defect, and at surgery, a bulging degenerated disc may be found, but not a truly "ruptured" disc. Removal of such a disc often fails to relief the patient's pain. It is estimated that 30–40% of the patients undergoing disc surgery fail to achieve complete pain relief [1, 2].

Pedersen, Blunck, and Gardner [8] performed anatomical studies of the articular nerve of Luschka in the lumbar spine. The posterior ramus leaves the lumbar nerve root just distal to the sensory ganglion, it passes inferiorly and dorsal through the intertransverse ligament and between the facet joint and the transverse process and sends branches into the articular capsule of the inferior facet.

Based on these studies Rees [9] passed transcutaneously a special tenotomy blade to the intertransverse ligament to section the nerve supplying the facets. He reported 99,8% success in treating 29 patients with low back and extremities pain, but he found a 20% incidence of subcutaneous hematoma.

Shealy [10, 11] changed the blind knife approach to a percutaneous temperature controlled radiofrequency electro-coagulation technique. He introduced this method of treatment in the United States.

More recently, Fox and Rizzoli [3] identified the radiological co-ordinates for the posterior articular nerve of Luschka in the lumbar spine.

The results obtained by these surgeons and those by Ouden-hoven [6] encouraged us to start doing this procedure in our patients.

Technique

Under fluoroscopic guidance a no. 19 gauge spinal needle, insulated to 8 mm from the tip is guided to the tender facet joint. The target point lies at the lower portion of the facet joints or between the lower portion of the facet joint and the projection of the pedicle on end [13].

The introduction of the needle can be done with the patient in the prone position and then is placed in the oblique position with the affected side 45° up and the X-ray tube vertically above, or the needle can be introduced with the pacient in the oblique position from the start. The oblique view is the most important to visualized the facet joint. A lateral view indicates the distance of the needle from the main nerve root.

Electrical stimulation (25 CPS, 1–2 volts) applied to the needle should reproduce, at least in part, the patient's pain pattern. The patient usually feels a tingling sensation irradiating to the buttock and limb, which rarely goes beyond the popliteal fossa. If this response is not achieved with 1–2 volts the needle should be repositioned. When the needle is too close to the main root, stimulation elicites severe radicular pain and/or muscle contractions in the extremity. Sometimes the direct mechanical stimulation with the needle reproduces the original patient's pain. Occasionally the pain is referred to the contralateral side.

When we are certain that the lesion can be made, the needle is connected with the unipolar coagulator (Bovie) set at 2, and a 5–10 seconds lesion is made. Then, we stimulate again to make sure that the nerve has been coagulated. The same procedure is repeated at all tender joints painful to finger pressure.

We have not used radiofrequency electrocoagulation as it has been described by others [3, 6, 10, 11].

Material

We have performed percutaneous facet rhizotomy in 30 patients; of these, 26 had had no previous surgical treatment of their low back and sciatic pain, and 4 had had previous laminectomy for disc removal.

The duration of pain prior to this procedure ranged from 3 months to 10 years (Table 1).

The pain was low back and sciatic in 27 patients (20 unilateral, 7 bilateral) and low back only in 3.

Table 1. *Duration of Pain*

3 months–1 year	7 p.
1 year–3 years	16 p.
3 years–6 years	5 p.
More than 6 years	2 p.

Table 2. *Results*

	Excellent	Good	Failure	Total
No previous surgery	12	10	4	26
Previous laminectomy	0	1	3	4
Total	12	11	7	30

The follow up period ranges from 3 to 9 months. Common physical findings were restricted back motion, facet tenderness, muscle spasm and restricted straight leg raising. None of the patients had motor weakness, 10 patients had hipesthesia, and the ankle jerk was absent in 5 patients.

The radiological findings ranged from no anomalies at all to varying degrees of hypertrophic changes, narrowing interspace, spina bifida and transitional vertebra. Radiculography showed a "bulging" disc in 8 patients.

Results

We classified the results as "excellent" when the patient had at least 95% pain relief and was able to return to his original occupational activity; "good" when he had mild low back pain but no extremity pain, and "failure".

The results are shown in Table 2. We obtained "satisfactory" results in 23 (76%) patients. Of the patients with previous laminectomy only one had partial pain relief.

All the patients in the successful groups except 2 had a positive response to electrical stimulation, while in only 2 cases of the "failure" group the response was positive (Table 3).

Five patients were reoperated. Two of them had had a 50% pain relief at the first operation and attained an "excellent" result with the second procedure. The other 3 patients had no improvements at all of their pain in either operation.

Of the 7 failures, 5 did not get any pain relief and the other 2 had an immediate 50% improvement but returned to preoperative levels one week and one month later respectively.

Five patients with a "bulging" disc had an "excellent" result, one had a "good" result and 2 were "failures".

Table 3. *Response to Stimulation*

Group	Positive	Negative	Total
Excellent	11	1	12
Good	10	1	11
Failure	2	5	7
Total	23	7	30

Discussion

The best results are obtained in patients without previous operation. In those the results were poorer as it has been already reported [6, 10, 11]. The duration of pain is important; we obtained better pain relief in the cases with a recent pain history than in those with long chronic pain.

When the painful facet joints have been coagulated the patient should be asked to get up and do some exercises, if the pain has gone away the procedure should be stopped; on the contrary, if they still feel pain, the facet joints above and below and sometimes contralateral should be coagulated.

We think that before attempting surgical disc removal, and in those patients who have not major neurological deficit, facet denervation by percutaneous termocoagulation should be tried. Their pain may be secondary to facet strain or arthritis. No complications have been found with this procedure.

The results can be probably improved with the use of radiofrequency.

References

1. Barr, J., Kubik, Molloy, M., McNeill, J., Riseborough, E. (1967), Evaluation of end results in treatment of ruptured lumbar intervertebral discs with protrusion of nucleus pulposus. Surgery *125*, 250.
2. Dunkerley, G. E. (1971), Clinical Review. The results of surgery for low back and leg pain due to presumptive prolapsed intervertebral disc. Postgraduate Med. J. *47*, 120.
3. Fox, J., Rizzoli, H. (1973), Identification of radiologic coordinates for the posterior articular nerve of Luschka in the lumbar spine. Surg. Neurol. *1*, 343.

4. Goldthwait, J. (1911), The lumbo-sacral articulation. An explanation of many cases of "lumbago", "sciatica" and paraplegia. Boston Med. Surg. J. *64*, 365.
5. Mixter, W., Barr, J. (1934), Rupture of the intervertebral disc with involvement of the spinal canal. N.E.J.M. *211*, 210.
6. Oudenhoven, R. (1974), Articular rhizotomy. Surg. Neurol. *2*, 275.
7. Patti, V. (1927), New conceptions in the pathogenesis of sciatic pain. Lancet *2*, 53.
8. Pedersen, H., Blunck, C., Gardner, E. (1956), The anatomy of lumbosacral posterior rami and meningeal branches of the spinal nerves (sinu-vertebral nerves). J. Bone Joint Surg. *38-A*, 377.
9. Rees, W. (1971), Multiple bilateral subcutaneous rhizolysis of segmental nerves in the treatment of the intervertebral disc syndrome. Anh. Gen. Prac. *26*, 126.
10. Shealy, C. (1972), Articular nerve of Luschka. Rhizotomy for back and leg pain. Presented at the seminar on dorsal column stimulation, Temple University Philadelphia, Pa., Sept. 23, 1972.
11. Shealy, C. (1974), Facets in back and sciatic pain. Minn. Med. *57*, 199.

Authors' address: Dr. G. Flórez, Servicio de Neurocirugia, Hospital "Princesa Sofia", Leon, Spain.

Acta Neurochirurgica, Suppl. 24, 73 (1977)

Stereotactic Surgery in Gilles de la Tourette Syndrome

E. de Divitiis, A. D'Errico, and A. Cerillo

Three young patients, two females and one male, presented the characteristic symptomatology of multiple tics, obsessive motor compulsions and coprolalia. This symptomatology was accentuated when the patients tried to control it, especially in public. The patients had been treated with psychotherapy without benefit.

Hassler and Dieckmann have advocated thalamotomy in three patients with Gilles de la Tourette syndrome, in the belief that the conditions was of obsessive type. In agreement with this pathogenetic interpretation we have carried out the same operations under local anaesthesia using a modified Leksell apparatus. The stereotactic atlases of Talairach and of Schaltenbrand and Bailey were used and the ventricular structures outlined by air and the DM and iLa nuclei destroyed by radiofrequency coagulation.

The first intervention was always in the right thalamus and produced a complete remission in two patients, whilst the third had a small reduction of the compulsive symptomatology. No ill effects were seen. The third patient returned after about nine months with the same pre-operative symptomatology. He then had a second contralateral intervention, after which the symptomatology remained unchanged. In the other two patients the complete remission lasted for over a year. The return of the typical symptoms of the Gilles de la Tourette syndrome followed a prolonged period of mental confusion in one patient; in the other it returned progressively over a period of some months and both patients refused the contralateral operation.

In our experience therefore this procedure is not successful in treating the Gilles de la Tourette syndrome.

Authors' address: Prof. E. de Divitiis, Clinica Neurochirurgia II Facoltà di Medicina, Policlinico a Cappella dei Cangiani, Napoli, Italy.

Section II

Techniques

Acta Neurochirurgica, Suppl. 24, 77—83 (1977)
© by Springer-Verlag 1977

Servicio de Neurocirugia, Hospital Clinico Universitario, Valencia, Spain

Tomography in Stereotaxis.
A New Stereoencephalotome Designed for this Purpose

J. L. Barcia-Salorio, J. Barberá, J. Broseta, and F. Soler

With 4 Figures

After twenty years of experience in stereotactic surgery, we have come to the conclusion that the calculation of the target point from the conventional pneumoencephalography, which is the most innocuous of the methods in use, has the following disadvantages: a) It is not always possible to see the ventricular structures of the midline, third and fourth ventricules and the aqueduct, with sufficient clarity and safety. b) There is considerable asymmetry between the two hemispheres of the patient's brain. This poses problems when the calculation of the lateral position of the target is based on medially situated points. c) The information on a spatial situation, size and shape of the basal nuclei is obtained from the stereotactic atlases. These are composed of brain sections which do not always correspond to the shape of the whole brain obtained by pneumoencephalography.

In view of all this, we have thought to applying tomography to stereotaxis, because, in our view it has the following advantages: a) It provides better and safer visualization of midline structures. b) It is possible to explore the structures of the selected hemisphere only. c) It is possible to make a precise comparison of the atlas brain section with its corresponding tomographic "slice".

In order to use this method we have designed a new stereo-encephalotome which has the following characteristics. It has been designed primarily to work with an apparatus of multiplane tomography and a TV monitor, but can be used with conventional radiography as well.

The stereoencephalotome consists of a square frame fixed to the skull by means of four sharp pointed screws. The frame must be placed in a plane as nearly parallel to the AC-PC line as possible. We use a TV monitor to do this properly.

In the frame are four movable calibrated arms (Fig. 1), each one having a perpendicular offshoot at its midpoint. The arms are used firstly to determine the path of the central X-ray beam and the correct placement of the apparatus in the anterior-posterior and lateral projections. This is done by causing one opposing pair of

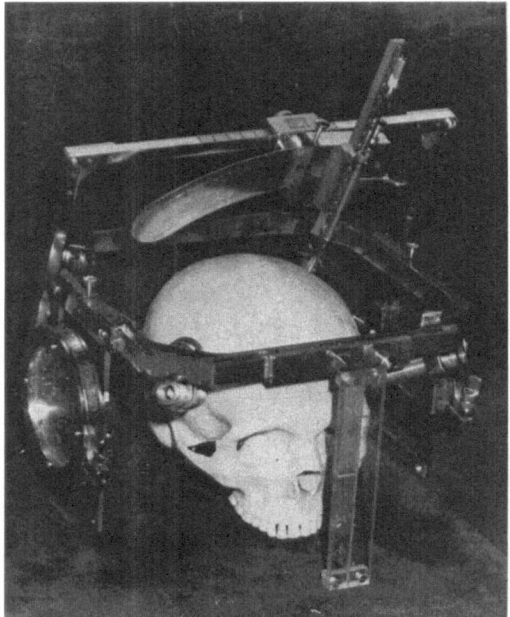

Fig. 1. See the text

arms to project so as to form a cross between them and their side-arms. Its second purpose is to fix the position of the target point in the three spatial dimensions (x, y, and z). The X-ray coordinates are determined by the same calibrated arms, which will frame the tomographic film; and, the z coordinates will be supplied by the graduated scale which shows the separation of the arms, and therefore the tomographic plane, with reference to the midline. Once the three cartesian coordinates of the target point have been decided, the calibrated arms are withdrawn. In their place a semiarc is fixed to the frame having on it an electrode carrier movable over the same arc. This electrode carrier is adjusted till its centre coincides with the target. The semiarc turns on the axis represented by the centre of the circular supports that hold it.

This stereoencephalotome being based on a radial system, the

electrode remains constantly directed at the target, independently
of the method of access decided. And this fact gives it great
versatility of use, allowing anterior approaches (orbital leucotomy,
transnasal hypophysectomy, etc.), posterior approaches (dentatectomy, etc.), lateral approaches (cervical cordotomy, tractotomy,

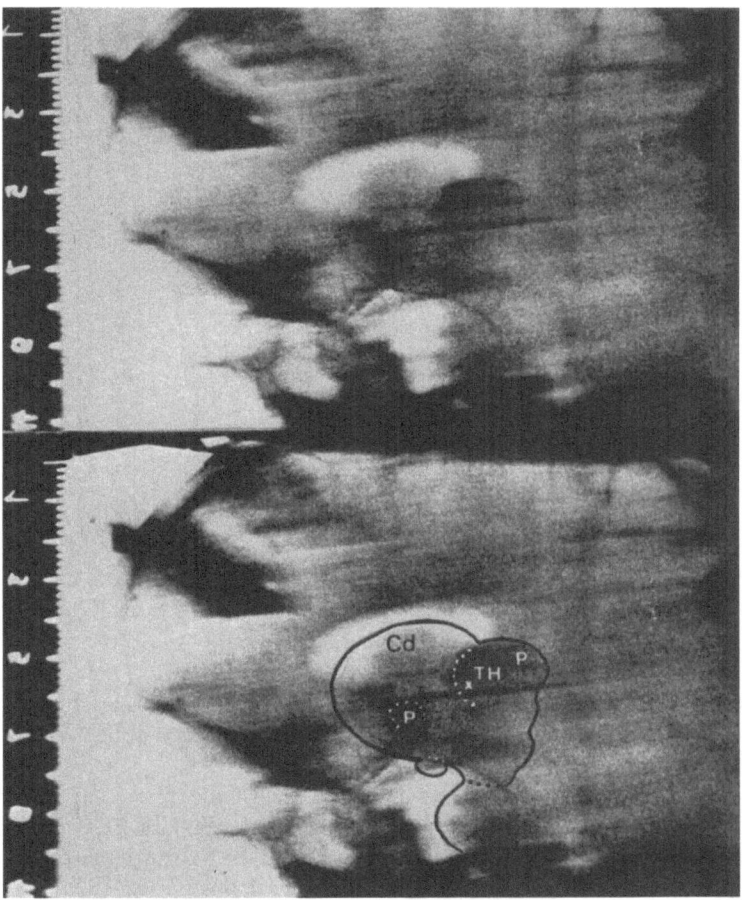

Fig. 2. Angiotomography made with our stereoencephalotome. Plane 10.5 mm.
On the left side it is possible to observe the calibrated arm. The thalamus, caudatus,
pallidum and nigral substance are visualized by the angiographic contrast in the
capillar phase. The internal capsula appears less vascularized

etc.) and from above as in thalamotomy, fornicotomy, amigdal-
otomy, etc., as well at its application to radiosurgery.

Surgical procedure with our apparatus is carried out as follows:

1. Targets Which are Visible Radiologically

In fornicotomy-anterior commisurotomy, etc., in which the target point is either itself visible or is in close relationship with a structure visible in the midline, the calibrated arms are placed on the 0 point or midline of the frame. Then, we carry out a tomographic section on this plane with the Princeps C.G.R., after having

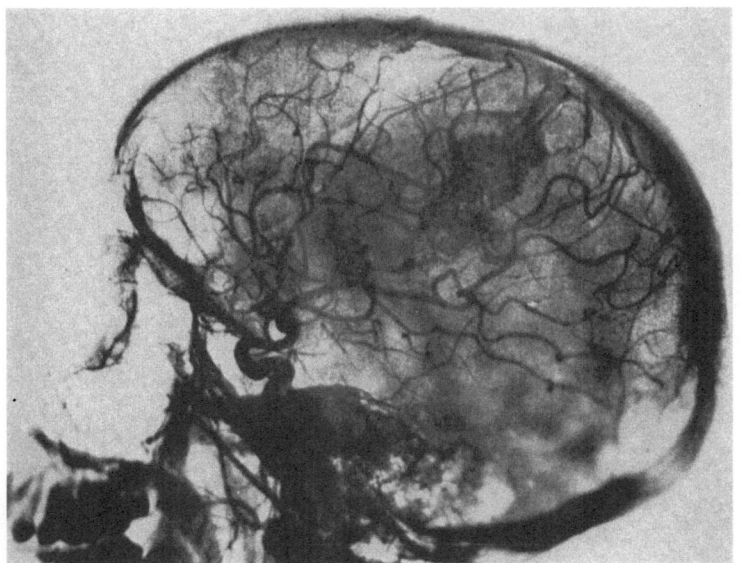

Fig. 3. Arteriovenous malformation. The nutrient artery can not be visualized because the high vascularization

injected air into the third and fourth ventricles. To control the accuracy of the tomographic section it must be possible to read the numbers on the arms on the X-ray film clearly.

Once the target point has been selected, it can be determinated by the two lines which cross over it and also intersect the two calibrated arms. Thus, the target has been fixed mathematically by four numbers. The translation of this calculation to the cartesian tridimensional system of the apparatus is made by means a nomogram.

When the electrode is placed on its support and guided to its calculated coordinates we can check the accuracy of our measurement with a radiograph in which both cross-wires representing the centre of the semiarc must fall on the selected target. The insertion of the electrode into the brain is then controlled by TV.

The advantages of our procedure are as follow: a) We have better visualization of the midline structures. b) It is possible to eliminate X-ray distortion because the target is in the same plane as the

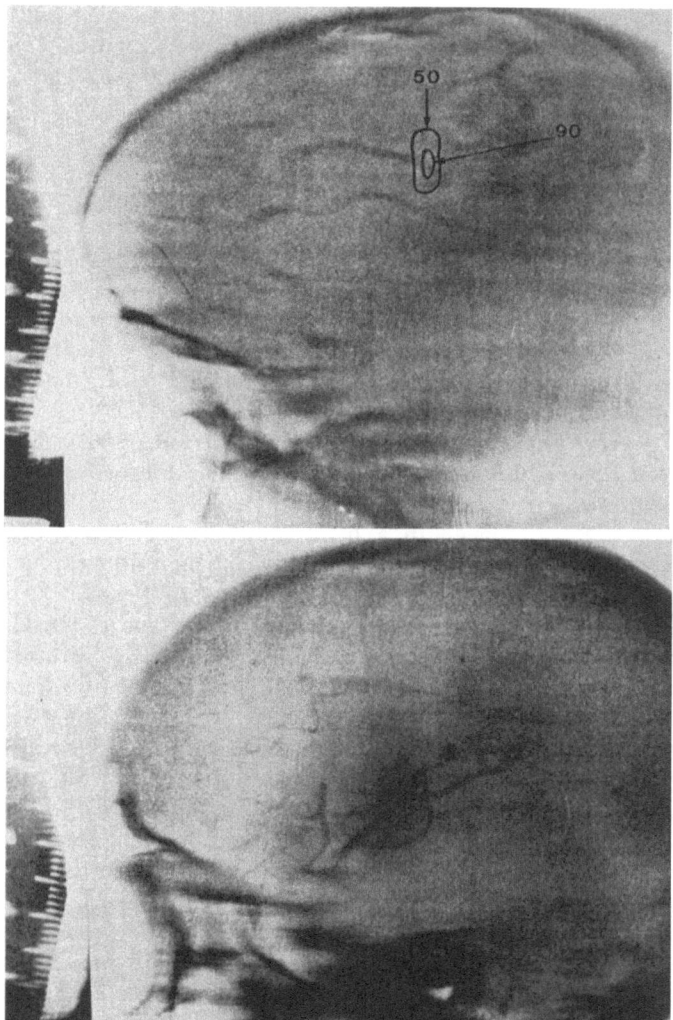

Fig. 4. By means of angiotomography the nutrient artery is better defined

calibrated arms. c) The system of two separated lines increases precision and decreases the chance of error (Dereymaeker *et al.* s/d).

d) There is preoperative control of the position of the electrode. And, e), the control of the electrode is monitored by TV.

2. *Targets Not Radiologically Visible Nor on the Midline*

In these cases angiopneumotomography is especially useful since the air images depict a great part of subcortical structures (caudatum, thalamus, hypothalamus, and chiasma) while the angiographic images especially in their capillary and early venous phases depict with sufficient accuracy those zones not seen by the air (Salomon 1971, Goldberg 1975). For this reason, we have found that the use of both techniques together with tomography provides a very good picture of basal structures.

On the other hand, we are very interested in the determination of the diencephalic profile, because one of us (Barcia-Salorio *et al.* 1969) has demonstrated that it is possible to correct with a high degree of precision any anatomic variations in a patient's brain in relation to the model of the atlas by means of a conformal mapping with an analogous field plotter.

We carry out tomography with the Princeps C.G.R. and a cassette-holder which allow us to get six simultaneous films with 5 mm separation between them.

The patient is placed in a head holder which has a graduated scale, marking each film the distance between the tomographic section and the midline, following the procedure of Goldberg (1975). After the injection of sufficient air into the ventricular and cisternal spaces, we make two monolateral carotid injections on the affected sides, calculating that the one tomographic shot can capture both capillary and arterial phases simultaneously (Fig. 2).

The diencephalic profiles thus obtained are fed by means of an XY plotter into a Digital PDF-8 e computer, to which we have previously fed the line drawings of the Schaltenbrand-Bailey (1959) atlas. Basing ourselves on the above mentioned paper of Barcia-Salorio *et al.* (1969), we have been able to digitalize the same geometrical transformation, which by comparing the corresponding profile of the plane from the atlas with that of the patient transfers the nuclei of the former to those of the latter. This process makes it possible to reproduce upon the screen of the display Tectronix 4010 the desired section of the brain with its principal nuclei depicted but now corresponding to those of the patient's brain, because the anatomic variations have been corrected by means a relaxation method.

Once, the target has been fixed and the way of approach decided on, we follow the stereotactic procedures as described above.

This procedure offers the following advantages: a) By the characteristics of the tomography, already described in the previous section, the X-ray distorsion is eliminated and direct calculation of the coordinates of the target point made possible. b) There is a better and more complete visualization of the diencephalic structures (Di Chiro 1961). c) The various anatomic and asymmetric variations are corrected, and d) as we are able to visualize the vessels near the target we can take steps to avoid a serious lesion in them.

Finally, as we have already stated, the radial position of the stereoencephalotome permits its application to radiosurgery, which we perform, according to Leksell (1951) the first procedure, connecting our apparatus to a source of Co^{60} Theratron 780 of the Atomic Energy of Canada, Ltd., equivalent to 1.27 Mev. and an output of 6,000 Ci. Putting circular diaphragms which reduce to 3.5 and 8 mm diameter of ionizing beam in a semiarc, we can make use of the well-known cross-fire method.

The advantages of our tomographic model in this case are: a) Better visualization of the lesions to be radiated. As instance, in the case of a arteriovenous malformation the nutrient artery is usually masked by other vessels (Fig. 3). With the angiotomography we can isolate the principal vessels in each plane (Goldberg 1975) (Fig. 4). b) In the radiosurgery of the trigeminal neuralgia or in hypophysectomy in which an exact bone reference is needed, tomography increases precision and ease of location and localization of the affected part.

References

Barcia-Salorio, J. L., Martinez Carrillo, J. A. (1969), Calculation of the target point by means of an analogue plotter. In: Third Symposium on Parkinson's disease, pp. 223—232 (Gillingham, F. J., Donaldson, I. M. I., eds.). London: Livingstone. Ed.

Dereymaeker, A., De Dobbeler (s/d), Contribución al progreso de la estereotaxia cerebral. Nuevo estereoencefalotomo humano. UTEC. Heverlee (Louvain).

Di Chiro, G. (1961), An atlas of detailed normalp neumoencephalographic anatomy. Springfield, Ill.: Ch. C Thomas.

Goldberg, H. I. (1975), Angiografia cerebral con amplificación y angiotomografia en los accidentes vasculares. In: Enfermedades vasculares cerebrales (McDowell, H. H., Brenan, R. W., eds.). Barcelona: Toray, S.A.

Leksell, L. (1951), The stereotactic method and radiosurgery of the brain. Acta. Chir. Scand. *102*, 316—319.

Salamon. G. (1971), Atlas de la vascularisation arterielle du cerveau chez l'home. Paris: Sandoz. Ed.

Schaltenbrand, G., Bailey, P. (1959), Introduction to stereotaxis with an atlas of human brain. Stuttgart: G. Thieme.

Authors' address: J. L. Barcia Salorio, M.D., *et al.*, Servicio de Neurocirugia Hospital Clinico Universitorio, Valencia, Spain.

Acta Neurochirurgica, Suppl. 24, 85—98 (1977)
© by Springer-Verlag 1977

Departments of Surgery, Physiology, and Electrical Engineering of the University
of Toronto and the Neurosurgical Division, Toronto General Hospital, U.S.A.

Computerized Graphic Display of Results
of Subcortical Stimulation During Stereotactic Surgery*

R. R. Tasker, P. Hawrylyshyn, I. H. Rowe, and L. W. Organ

With 9 Figures

Summary

An on-line computer programme is described and illustrated which is capable
of displaying graphically in the form of Woolsey-type figurine charts stimulation-
induced responses obtained during stereotactic surgery. Not only can these data
then be optimally utilized for lesion localization but also the programme includes
facilities for a variety of types of analysis of the tape-stored data pooled from
all patients studied.

Introduction

Recent advances in the biomedical applications of computer
technology have ushered in a new phase of stereotactic surgery. The
capability of contemporary computers for graphic display has
already been exploited in many centres to allow the neurosurgeon
to follow the progress of a stereotactic probe through successive
brain structures. Over the past two years we have developed and
refined an on-line computer system which combines with these
anatomical capabilities the graphic display of the physiological data
collected optimizing their use in the search for the ideal lesion site.
The inclusion of a facility for data storage and for selective display
of pooled material from all patients has given us a unique tool for
the further refinement of stereotactic surgery and for the study of the
functional organization of the human brain stem.

Stereotactic Method

Stereotactic procedures, all performed for the relief of intractable
pain or involuntary movement, are carried out with the authors'
method [1] in two stages using the Leksell frame. During the first

---

* Supported by grants from The Toronto General Hospital Foundation.

stage, a positive contrast third ventriculogram permits measurement of three dimensional frame coordinates for the anterior and posterior commissures, for a third point on the mid-sagittal plane of the brain, usually the top of the septum pellucidum, and, if desired, of the dorsal height of the thalamus. During the second stage, performed

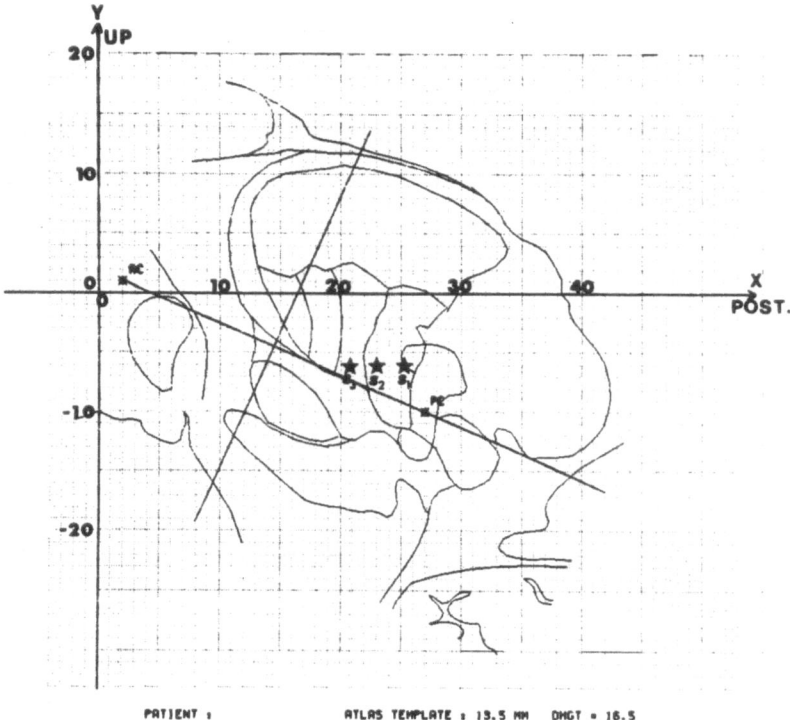

Fig. 1. Computerized brain template obtained by adjusting the 13.5 mm lateral sagittal diagram from the Schaltenbrand and Bailey atlas to the patient's brain dimensions plotted in terms of stereotactic frame coordinates. Stars mark sites chosen for exploration. *AC, PC, DHGT* indicate respectively anterior commissure, posterior commissure, and dorsal height of thalamus

under local anaesthesia, threshold stimulation is carried out with a bipolar 1.1 mm concentric electrode with an 0.5 mm pole separation using trains of 60 to 100 Hz biphasic 3 mS square waves. The burr hole is so placed that the electrode advances parasagittally as stimulation is carried out every 2 mm from 10 mm above to 10 to 16 mm below three target sites 2 mm apart in the same sagittal plane selected on the basis of the X-ray studies. The threshold responses

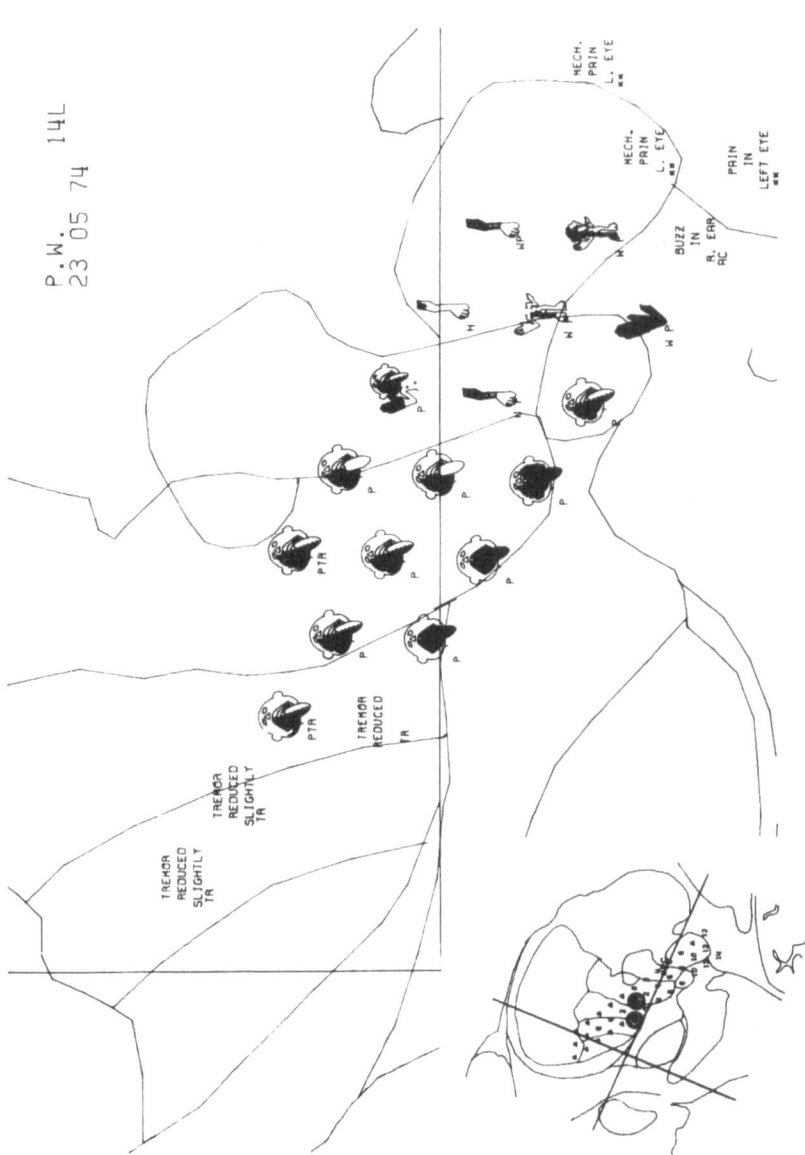

Fig. 2. Computer-plotted left-side brain template (insert) and figurine chart at 14 mm from the midline for patient P. W. with Parkinson's disease. TR, P, W, H, AC indicate respectively stimulation-induced tremor reduction, paresthesiae, warmth, hot, contralateral auditory response. Stars on template indicate lesion sites. See text for further explanation

are graphically plotted on-line by the computer in the form of Woolsey-type figurine charts.

Computer Technique

To display the data a Tektronix 4013 graphics display terminal is located in the operating room interfaced by telephone with an IBM 370-165 computer. The terminal is operated under an interactive version of Fortran and employs graphics software routines compatible with a Gould 5000 electrostatic plotter and a Calcomp incremental pen plotter.

At the end of the first stage of the stereotactic procedure the computer plots on paper an operative template as shown in Fig. 1 in readiness for selection of tentative targets for exploration during the second stage. The appropriate sagittal section from the Schaltenbrand and Bailey [2] atlas is stretched or shrunk as need be along the intercommissural line and, if desired, dorsoventrally, until it fits the patient's brain dimensions. The resultant atlas template is then plotted with a superimposed grid ruled in millimeters and reading in Leksell frame coordinates. Using the data supplied the computer can correct for any malposition of the stereotactic frame from a true midsagittal position with respect to the brain.

Storage of the physiological data evoked during the second stage of the procedure is accomplished with reference to numbered homonculus diagrams divided into numbered body regions. In addition, alphanumeric symbols indicate the quality of somatosensory response such as tingling and coolness and the presence of auditory, vestibular, visual or other effects. At the start of the second stage the atlas template corresponding to the sagittal section containing the proposed electrode tracts is plotted on the terminal screen in the operating room. Then as each site is stimulated, the required homunculus diagram appears on the screen appropriately positioned with the body part to which any somatosensory response is referred shaded in along with symbols indicating other information. In this manner it is possible to study the anatomical relationships of the physiological data, particularly the patterns of somatotopographic organization of the somatosensory system for the purpose of selection of lesion sites.

Results

On the basis of over 130 computer-plotted stereotactic procedures it has been possible to trace the primary sensory pathways (auditory, vestibular, visual, lemniscal, and spinothalamic) coursing through the midbrain and thalamus. The pattern of responses presented in Fig. 2

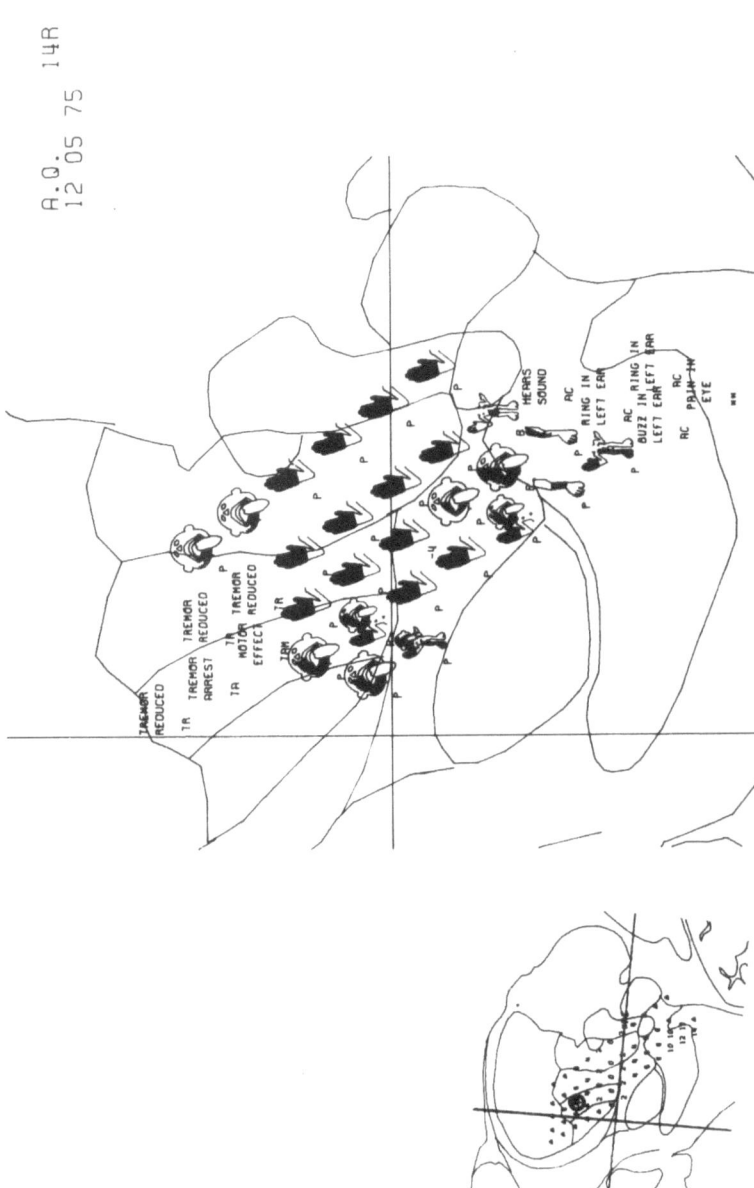

Fig. 3. As in Fig. 2 but a different Parkinsonian patient stimulated on the right side. Plotting is conventionally shown as for the left side of brain. In addition to symbols used in Fig. 2, *TA, M, B* indicate respectively stimulation-induced tremor arrest, motor response, and burning. Note that in contrast to Fig. 2 the physiological data do not fit the atlas template for they and accordingly the "successful" lesion site are all displaced superoanteriorly. This exemplifies the importance of on-line inspection of graphically displayed physiological data during stereotactic surgery

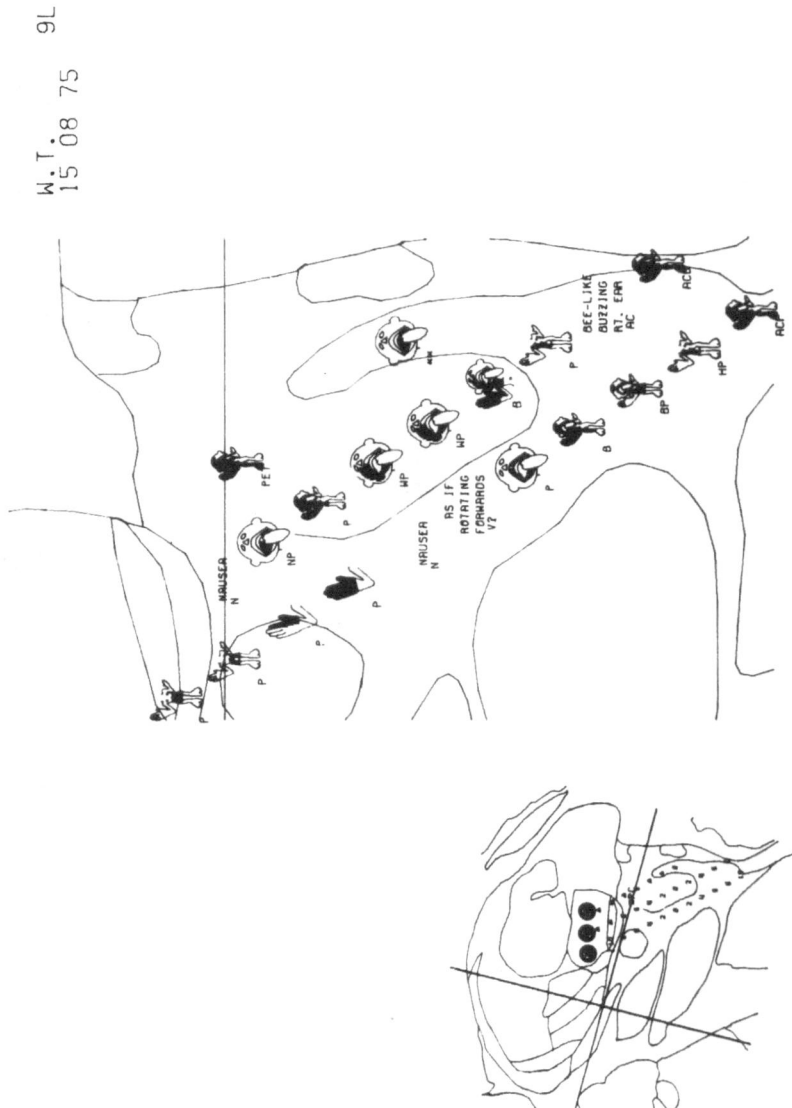

Fig. 4. Computerized plot as in Fig. 2 in patient W. T. with intractable pain at 9 mm from midline. *N, V, E* indicate respectively stimulation-induced nausea, vertigo, emotional disturbance. The interrelationships of lemniscal, spinothalamic, and auditory pathways are shown

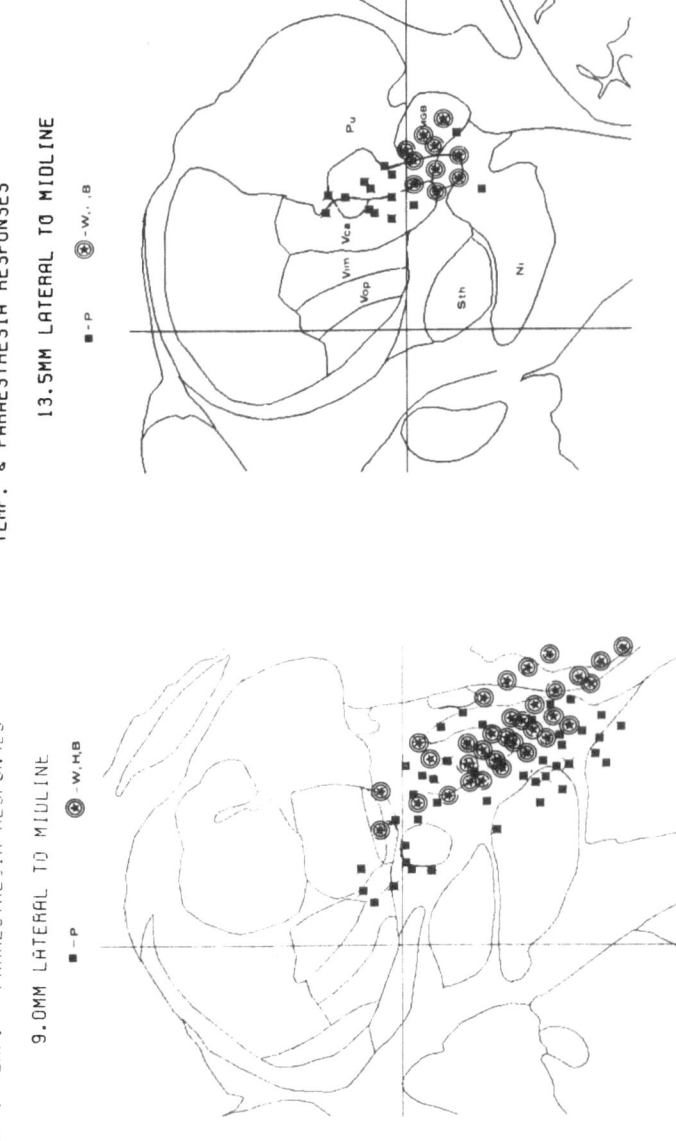

Fig. 5. Computerized "search-and-plot" diagram of all paraesthetic and temperature coded responses from 130 patients elicited by stimulation at 9 mm (left) and 13.5 mm (right) from the midline. The more dorsal position of the temperature-coded responses is in keeping with their origin in the spinothalamic tract which lies dorsally adjacent to the medial lemniscus in the midbrain and relays in the thalamus posterior to the lemniscal relay in the main portion of the ventrobasal complex. P indicates stimulation-induced paraesthesia, arising in the lemniscal pathway, WHB warm hot or burning, originating in the lateral spinothalamic pathway

typifies stimulation of the brain stem 14 mm from the midline. The paraesthetic face responses constitute the facial part of the thalamic homunculus for the medial lemniscus organized somatotopographically from 10 to 18 mm from the midline where stimulation gives rise to a feeling of tingling, shock or vibration solely on the contralateral side of the body. However, contiguously posteroinferiorly there is a somatotopographic discontinuity with trunk and leg responses representing stimulation of the spinothalamic tract. Here between 14 and 17 mm from the midline, responses are usually described as warm or cool tingling, occasionally burning or pain, they occasionally involve the ipsilateral as well as the contralateral half of the body, and are somatotopographically dorsoventrally organized [3].

Immediately posteroinferior to the thalamic relay of the spino-thalamic tract is seen a site where stimulation elicits buzzing in the contralateral ear, representing activation of the auditory pathway whose chiefly contralateral responses can be traced through the lateral lemniscus immediately dorsal to the spinothalamic tract in the midbrain through the brachium of the inferior colliculus to the medial geniculate [4]. Though not occurring in this particular patient, stimulation adjacent to the auditory pathway often elicits a sense of rotation or movement indicating activation of the vestibular pathway. In some patients such responses are also found in the sub-thalamus and just anterior to the ventrobasal complex. The double asterisks indicate ipsilateral head pain arising from mechanical and/or electrical stimulation of the pial surface of the brain stem, their location closely fitting that predicted by the atlas template. Stimulation superoanterior to the lemniscal responses reduced, and a lesion here abolished, this Parkinsonian patient's hand tremor.

Fig. 3 illustrates the mapped responses obtained by stimulation 14 mm from the midline in another Parkinsonian patient. In contrast to the patient in Fig. 2, the physiological map is shifted 3 to 5 mm superoanteriorly compared with the atlas template based on the radiological studies, so that, had not the lesion been similarly displaced, it would not have been successful in arresting the patient's tremor. Fig. 3 illustrates the importance of on-line inspection of graphically displayed physiological data in stereotactic surgery. The predominance of lemniscal hand responses seen in Fig. 3 suggests a more lateral position in the homunculus than that displayed in Fig. 2.

During 32 stereotactic procedures performed for the relief of intractable pain, stimulation of the upper midbrain between 5 and 12 mm from the midline presents a picture analogous to that reported above. Fig. 4 illustrates the data obtained by stimulating the left midbrain of patient W. T. at 9 mm from the midline. Anteriorly stimulation induced at low threshold a contralateral feeling of tingling at sites which coincide with the course of the medial lemniscus. Stimulation dorsal to these sites induces not a feeling of

SAGITTAL PLANE AT : 13.5 MM.

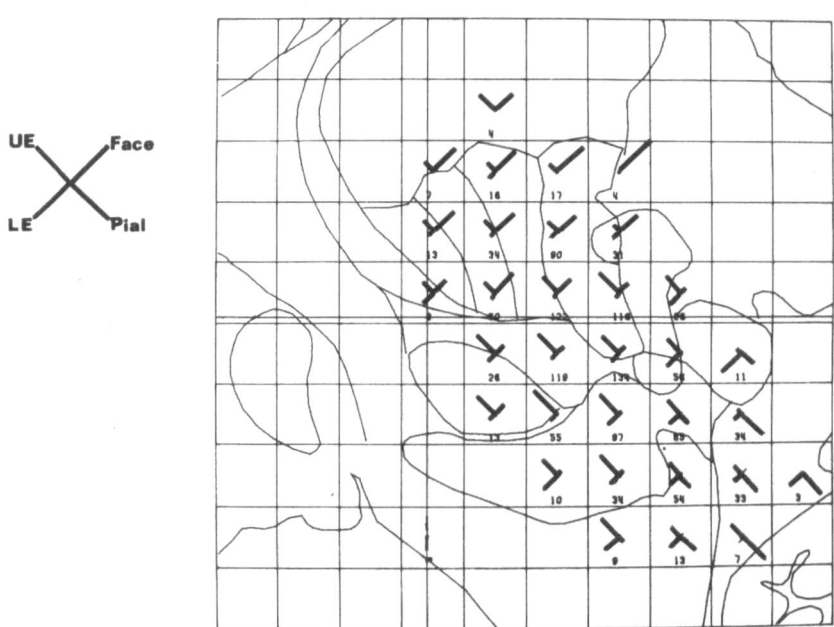

Fig. 6. Computerized analysis of all 1,265 sites stimulated in 130 patients at 14 mm from the midline. The atlas template is broken down into square cells, the number of responses in each of which is indicated by arabic numerals. These data are then analyzed for the percentage of responses reported in face, upper extremity, lower extremity, and ipsilateral head (indicating pial stimulation) respectively, the actual percentages being shown by the length of diagonals to the upper right, upper left, lower left, and lower right respectively. The preponderance of pial responses along the dorsal margin of the brain stem posterioinferiorly as well as that of leg responses arising from stimulation of the spinothalamic tract immediately subjacent to the pia is well shown. Facial and upper limb responses are mostly derived from stimulation of the lemniscal relay of the ventrobasal complex

tingling but rather a warm or hot tingling or burning at sites where spinothalamic fibres are located. Immediately dorsal to such responses again, auditory and often vestibular responses from the lateral lemniscus and brachium of inferior colliculus are identified just deep

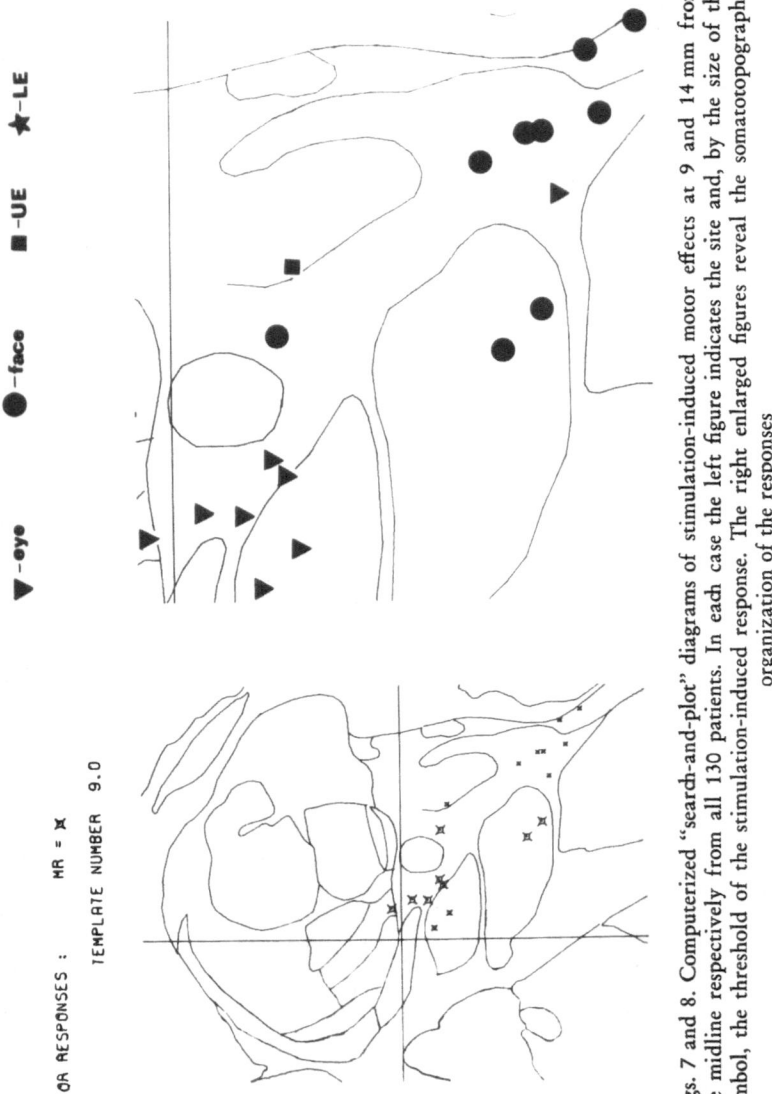

Figs. 7 and 8. Computerized "search-and-plot" diagrams of stimulation-induced motor effects at 9 and 14 mm from the midline respectively from all 130 patients. In each case the left figure indicates the site and, by the size of the symbol, the threshold of the stimulation-induced response. The right enlarged figures reveal the somatotopographic organization of the responses

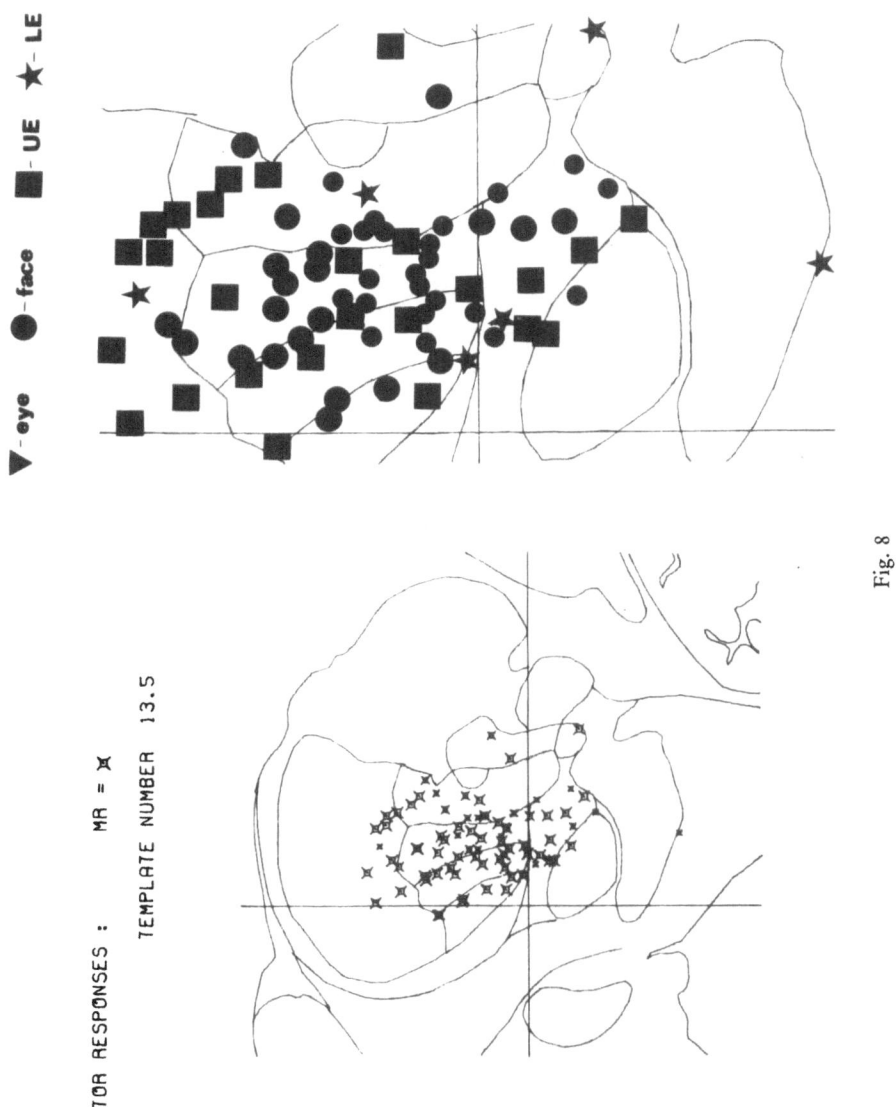

Fig. 8

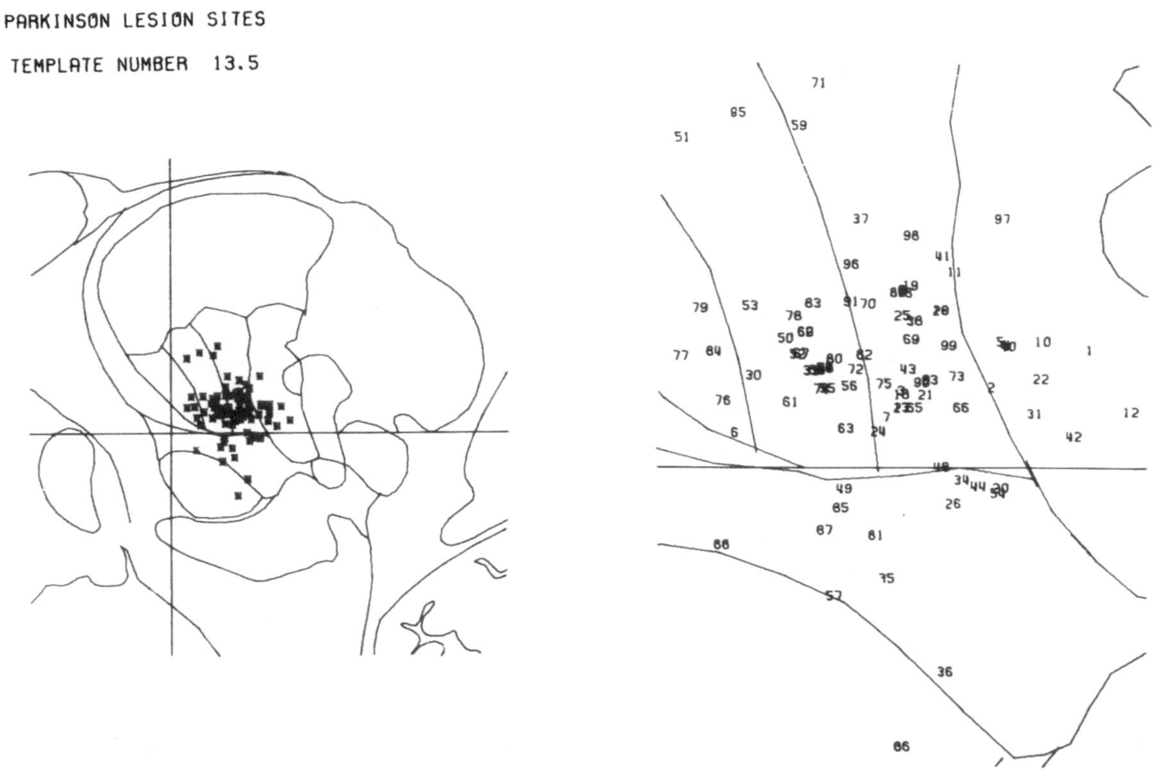

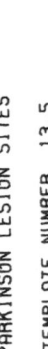

PARKINSON LESION SITES

TEMPLATE NUMBER   13.5

Fig. 9. Computerized "search-and-plot" diagram for all lesions made for the control of Parkinsonian tremor at 14 mm from the midline in all 130 patients. The enlarged right figure identifies the patients by numerals which refer to data in hard copy

to the pial surface. From these examples it can be seen how the computer-plotted display of physiological data optimizes their use through visual inspection for the selection of lesion sites.

The operative and physiological data from over 130 stereotactic cases have been stored on computer tape allowing the pool of data from all patients to be scanned for any chosen type of response. Fig. 5 shows a cumulative plot of contralateral paraesthetic versus temperature-coded responses. Again it can be noted that the para-esthetic responses representing medial lemniscal stimulation are positioned generally ventral to the temperature-coded responses representing spinothalamic sites. In plotting such responses, the computer corrects for variations in intercommissural distances between patients by conforming their location to the standard atlas template.

Fig. 6 shows another approach to analyzing pooled physiological data. The atlas template is broken down into square cells and all stimulation sites from the 130 patients falling in a particular cell are collectively examined. The computer determines the fraction of responses in the cell which were facial, upper extremity, lower extremity or pial in nature and plots these percentages along the appropriate diagonals whose complete length represents 100%. From the 1,265 sites examined the ventrodorsal transition from facial and upper extremity lemniscal responses to leg responses of the spino-thalamic relay and pial stimulation sites becomes apparent.

In addition to comparing response regions, this search-and-plot facility is capable of selecting stimulation sites exhibiting any of 30 qualities of response codes. Figs. 7 and 8 identify sites with stimulation-induced motor effects. At 9 mm from the midline the cluster of ocular sites reflects stimulation of the oculomotor nerve while the more inferior and dorsal limb responses probably reflect activation of cerebral peduncle. At 13 mm lateral, motor responses are clustered largely anterior to the ventrobasal complex where the greatest concentration of somatosensory responses occur as shown in Fig. 8. It is thought that these responses arise from stimulation of the motor thalamus (ventrolateral nucleus).

The computer can also plot lesion sites for all patients with a particular diagnosis as illustrated in Fig. 9. For Parkinson's disease the lesions are concentrated along the rostral margin of the ventro-basal nucleus. From such plots the clinical effectiveness of lesions can be correlated with their location.

References

1. Tasker, R. R., Organ, L. W. (1972), Mapping of the somatosensory and auditory pathways in the upper midbrain and thalamus in man. In: Neurophysiology

studied in man, pp. 169—187 (Somjen, G. G., ed.). Amsterdam: Excerpta Medica.
2. Schaltenbrand, G., Bailey, P. (1959), Introduction to stereotaxis with an atlas of the human brain. Stuttgart: G. Thieme.
3. Emmers, R., Tasker, R. R. (1975), The human somesthetic thalamus. New York: Raven Press.
4. Tasker, R. R., Organ, L. W. (1973), Stimulation-mapping of the human upper auditory pathway. J. Neurosurg. *38*, 320—325.

Authors' address: R. R. Tasker, M.D., F.R.C.S., Room UWI-124, Toronto General Hospital, Toronto MG5 IG7, Canada.

Acta Neurochirurgica, Suppl. 24, 99—10? (1977)

Department of Stereotactic Neurosurgery and Neuronuclear Medicine,
Neurosurgical University Hospital, Freiburg i. Br., Federal Republic of Germany

A Computer Programme System
for Stereotactic Neurosurgery*

W. Birg, F. Mundinger, and M. Klar

With 9 Figures

Summary

A computer programme system is reported which allows a simulation
of a stereotactic operation. It incorporates the determination of intracerebral
structures and the electrode tract by means of bony reference points as well as
the calculation of the parameters for the stereotactic apparatus.

It contains further a library of brain sections, by which the electrode tract
within the target structures can be shown on a computer display.

Key words: Brain, computer, stereotactic operation, graphic representation,
brain atlas.

Introduction

The advantages of employing the computer in stereotactic brain
operations [7] are becoming more and more evident [2, 9, 11]. The result
is maximal accuracy, better results and a further reduction in risks.
Our stereotactic target apparatus was first modified for computer
calculation three years ago. Since then, it has brought excellent
results for the last 700 of our total of 5,200 stereotactic operations.

Today we can present a complete computer programme system
that even permits a simulation of the operation before the first
incision.

Programme Description

As the flow chart shows (Fig. 1) the programme system consists
mainly of two modules, a target point programme which permits
calculation of intracerebral structures by means of the skull coordinates on the X-ray pictures [6, 8] and the angle parameters for the

---

* With the support of the special research division—brain research and
physiology of the senses (SFB 70 E 2) of the Deutsche Forschungsgemeinschaft.

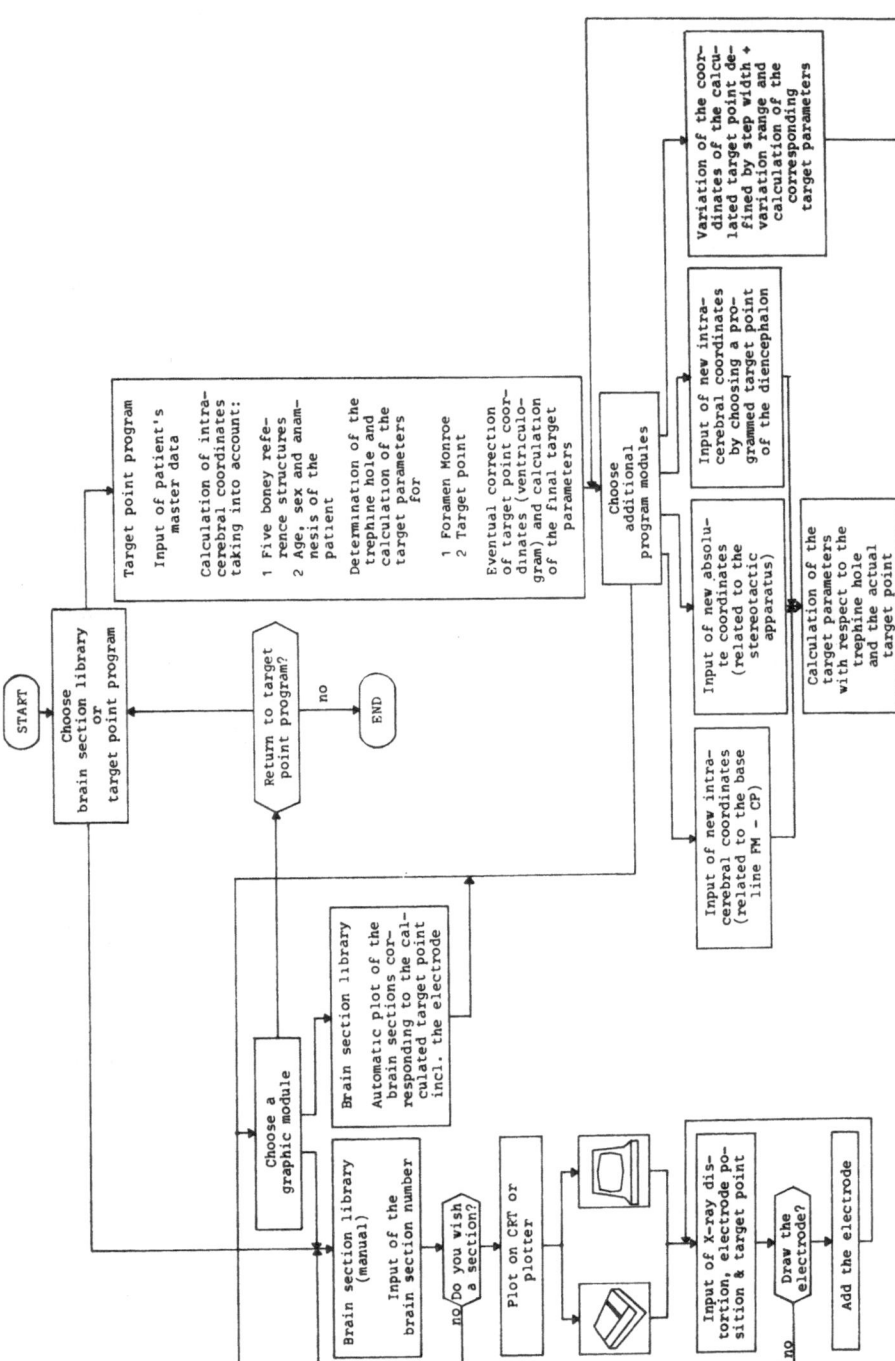

Fig. 1. Flow chart of the neurosurgical programme system

stereotactic apparatus [4], and a graphic programme which performs the drawing of relevant brain sections on a graphic computer display.

This programme system may be illustrated with the following example:

Once the base system of the stereotactic apparatus has been attached to the patients head and primary X-rays have been made in two planes, four boney reference points (Fig. 2) are determined.

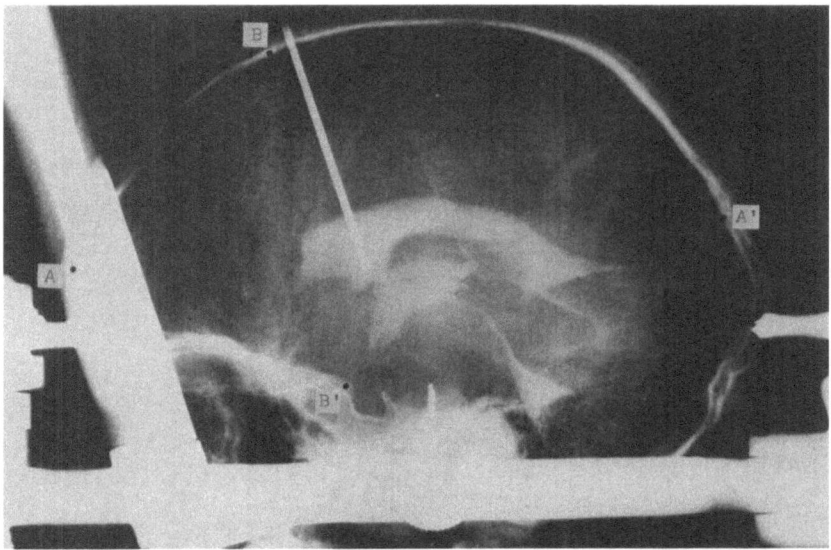

Fig. 2. Boney reference points on the X-ray. *A* Point of intersection for the squama frontalis and the partes ossis frontalis on the tabula interna, *A'* point of intersection of the lambda suture on the tabula interna, or the tip of the os interparietale, *B* point of intersection of the coronal suture on the tabula interna (= bregma), *B'* interclinoidal point, *i.e.*, the interpolation between the anterior clinoid processes of the sella at the transition to the tuberculum sellae. The target point (entry of Foramen Monroe) has been calculated by means of cranio-cerebral relations for the positive contrast ventriculography. The probe is situated in the target point, the ventricular system is visible in all parts

These reference points have a phylogenetic correlation [8] to the main axis of the brain (Foramen Monroe—commissura posterior). The input of their coordinates is still made by the terminal keyboard; meanwhile we are working on a programme which will enable us to use a light pen for the input of these coordinates.

When these values have been ascertained, the basic data for the patient are fed into the computer. These data include: earlier operation, the hemisphere of the operative intervention and the X-ray distortion (Fig. 3).

Subsequently we feed in the data corresponding to the projected angle of penetration for the electrode, *e.g.*, 65 degrees from the intracerebral base line (Foramen Monroe—commissura posterior) and 10 degrees from the medial plane and further the hemisphere co-ordinates for the A.P.-reference.

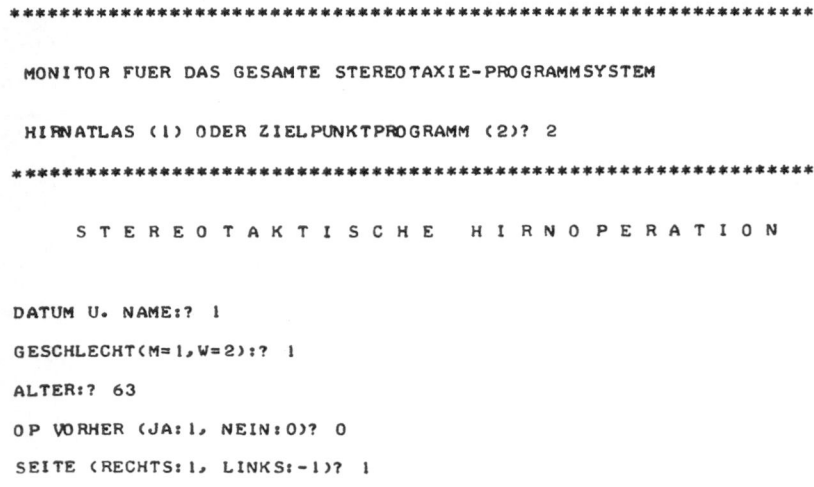

Fig. 3
Figs. 3–7. Programme dialogue with operator

Then the intracerebral coordinates of the target point are fed in. For the present example—a subthalamotomy—these coordinates are for the zona incerta 8 mm laterally of the border of the third ventricle (Sulcus interventriculare), 12 mm posterior of the caudal and ventral border of Foramen Monroe and 6 mm ventrally of the base line. If the calcification of the Pinealis is visible, its coordinates are measured, too (Fig. 4).

Now the coordinates of FM and CP are calculated by the computer, based on 14,000 cranio-cerebral data taken from 430 pneum-encephalograms, that have been made for former stereotactic operations. For our example: the upper entrance at the left of FM for guided positive contrast myelography using 2 cm³ of Dimer-X®. We then await the automatic calculation of the trepanation point on the skull with the question: "Trepanation point O.K.?" Here it is possible to make a desired change, for example, in case of a particular shape of the skull or to avoid pacchionic granulations, etc. (Fig. 5).

```
    RS      RA         ROENTGENVERZEICHNUNG
  ? 10.75, 10.84


    WS      WA         WINKEL  SAG  U.  AP
  ? 65,     10


    XR      XL         AP-HEMISPHAERENKOORDINATEN
  ? 80,    -78


    U    V    W        INTRACEREBRALKOORDINATEN
  ? 8,  12,  -6


         Y  UND  Z-KOORDINATEN  DER  SCHAEDELREFERENZPUNKTE:


           S                  K
  ? 100,       50,       50,     125


           L                  I
  ? -80,       90,       23,     29


           P                  PINEALIS: WENN UNSICHTBAR: 0,0
  ?   0,       0
```

Fig. 4

```
    SL= 184.39      KI= 99.72        SL/KI= 1.85

    ROE: K1= 78.04        K4= 31.17

                         X              Y             Z

    ROE: FM            3.38          22.63         60.17

    PAT: FM            3.12          21.05         55.97

  ? 1

    ROE: TP           25.79          46.06         125

    PAT: TP           23.79          42.85         116.28


     TREPANATIONSPUNKT O.K.  ( JA: 1, NEIN: 0 ) :? 1

    ROE: TP           25.79          46.06         125

    PAT: TP           23.79          42.85         116.28

  ? 1
```

Fig. 5

For the target "Foramen Monroe" the computer now gives us the parameters to adjust the stereotactic apparatus: angle of elevation, lateral angle, vertical and lateral angles of rotation for the electrodes and the depth of the probe. After each parameter calculation an electronic phantom test is performed, *i.e.*, back-calculation to the target point coordinates. Additionally, the actual target point, in the present case zona incerta, will be printed. Eventually, its

coordinates are ascertained by a following ventriculography (Fig. 6).
Large nuclei such as cingulum, pulvinar or the sensomotorical nuclei
can be determined with sufficient accuracy without any ventriculogram, if the cranial reference points are such, that the calculated
coordinates fall within the range of a standard deviation of 1.5 mm
from the true value. If this precision cannot be attained, a ventriculography is necessary.

```
###########################################################

              PARAMETER FUER DAS ZIELGERAET

 SW              HW              NS              NV              NT
 79.82           67.38           1.21            4.1             165.54


=> ZP            ZX= 12.16       ZY= 9.58        ZZ= 50.33

###########################################################

PAT: BASISLAENGE = 22.12
     <) ZWISCHEN BASIS UND S-L: 63.23

   FS  CS  XM     VENTRIKULOGRAPHIE: FM,  CP,  MITTELLINIE
? 1,60,20,64,0

                 X               Y               Z

ROE: ZP          12.18           12.03           55.73

PAT: ZP          11.24           11.19           51.84

? 1
```

Fig. 6

If the ventricle is filled, then the definitive coordinates for the
FM, CP, and the new medial plane—provided the latter has been
transposed with respect to the cranial plane of symmetry by pathological changes—must be fed into the computer (Fig. 6). On the basis
of these values the final target is determined and is read out of the
computer together with the corresponding parameters for the stereotactic apparatus.

At this moment the operator has the choice between the following
programme modules (Fig. 1):

A. He can feed in new intra-cerebral coordinates (related to the
base line FM–CP) and repeat the calculation of the target parameters.

B. Instead of intra-cerebral, absolute coordinates (related to the
stereotactic apparatus) can be used.

3

ZIELPUNKT-BIBLIOTHEK:

ZONA INCERTA	DORSOMED. K.	PALLIDUM	V. PC. I.	V.O.A.
1	2	3	4	5
V.O.P.	LAMELLA MED.	NUCL. RUBER	NUCL. INT	PYRAM. I. IC
6	7	8	9	10
CAUDATUM K.	SENS. S. R.	NUCL. LIM.	V.C.PC. B	V.C.PC. A
11	12	13	14	15

ZIELPUNKT-NR.:? 1

U = 8   V = 12   W =-6   (INTRACEREBRAL-K)

X   Y   Z

ROE: ZP	12.18	12.03	55.73
PAT: ZP	11.24	11.19	51.84

? 1

Fig. 7

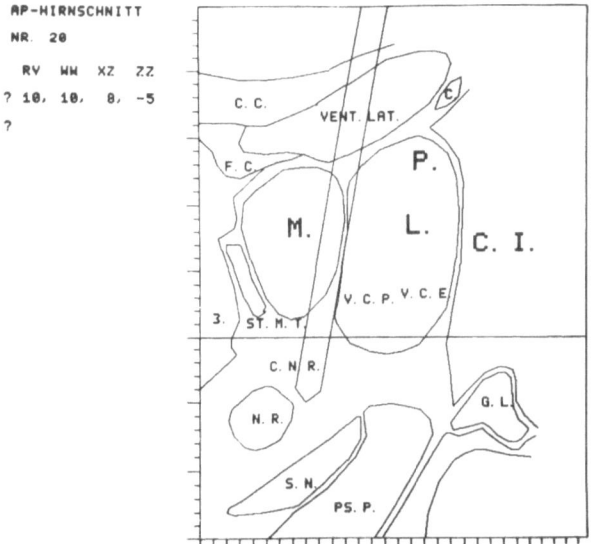

AP-HIRNSCHNITT
NR. 20

RV WW XZ ZZ
? 10, 10, 8, -5

?

Fig. 8. A "page" of the programmed brain atlas

C. Furthermore the neurosurgeon has a target point library at his disposal, by means of which he can choose programmed structures in the diencephalon (Fig. 7).

D. By means of a variation programme, finally the operator can vary systematically the target point coordinates within a cubic region and with arbitrary step width. So he has the possibility to perform small modifications of the electrode position independently from the computer.

The calculations concerning the target point being terminated, a graphic representation of the target structures on a computer display can be obtained. To that intention the corresponding pro-

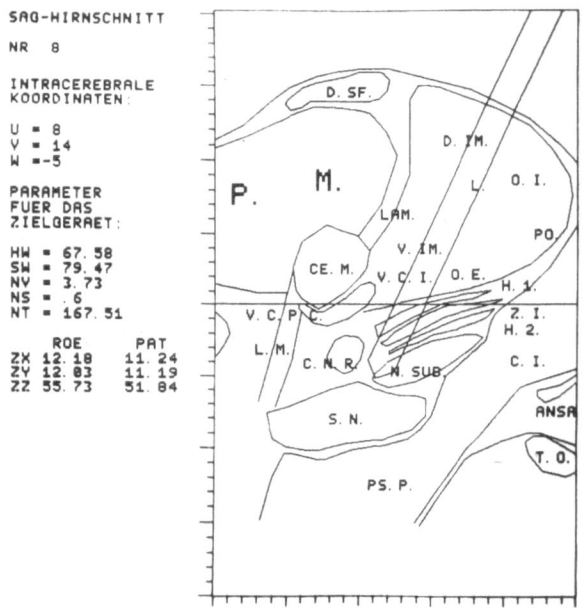

Fig. 9. An automatic plot of a brain section concerning the calculated target structure

gramme module contains a brain section library, here taken from the atlas by Andrew and Watkins [1].

This library can be used in two ways:

A. First the neurosurgeon can "read" in it like in an atlas, having the additional advantage, that the coagulation electrode can be drawn at the true scale and for an arbitrary target point and penetration angle (Fig. 8). The library actually contains 15 sagittal and 20 A.P. brain sections.

B. If it is desired, both the brain sections corresponding to the calculated target point can be drawn automatically. Each section then contains apart from the graphic representation the following additional information:

The section number, the intra-cerebral coordinates, in our example for zona incerta, and the corresponding angle parameters for the stereotactic apparatus as well as the absolute coordinates of the target point for the patient and for the X-ray picture (Fig. 9).

Again the representation of the brain section on the screen shows also the sheath of the electrode (diameter of 2 mm), which is introduced with a penetration angle of 65 degrees to the base line and 10 degrees from the median plane.

If the operator is satisfied with access and target point, he can go back to the target point programme. As in this case, generally each programme module can be obtained from each other, a feature which contributes to the flexibility of the programme system.

Conclusion

The surgical procedure does not begin until the whole intervention has been simulated on the computer terminal. The coagulation with the side-protruding electrode can equally be calculated by a programme, taking into account the electrode's position relative to the stereotactic apparatus [3].

This programme system enables us to avoid a possible risks, e.g., by modifying the penetration angle or by changing the trephine hole, for punctures of the diencephalon or the mid brain.

In conclusion we should like to mention that we are planning the complete programming of the Parkinson brain drawn by Hassler [5], which you will find in a monograph to be published shortly by the authors, and of the sections taken from the atlas of Schaltenbrand and Bailey [10]. We have also begun transferring the electrophysiological stimulation, stimuli control and coagulation to a process computer. With this the patient will be able to perform his own stimulation and we shall be able to study the bio-feedback mechanism involved in stereotactic brain operations.

References

1. Andrew, J., Watkins, E. S. (1969), A stereotaxic atlas of the human. Baltimore, USA.
2. Birg, W., Mundinger, F. (1973), Computer Calculations of target parameters for a stereotactic apparatus. Acta Neurochir. (Wien) 29, 123—129.
3. Birg, W., Mundinger, F. (1975), Calculation of the position of a side-protruding electrode tip in stereotactic brain operation using a stereotactic with polar coordinates. Acta Neurochir. (Wien) 32, 83—87.
4. Birg, W., Mundinger, F. (1974), Computer programs for stereotactic neurosurgery. Confin. Neurol. (Basel) 36, 326—333.
5. Hassler, R., Mundinger, F., Riechert, T., Parkinson syndrome in stereotaxis. Berlin-Heidelberg-New York: Springer. (In Press.)

6. Hoefer, Th., Mundinger, F., Reinke, M., Fuhrmann, G., Birg, W., Die computerunterstützte Berechnung subkortikaler Zielpunkte mit Hilfe der Röntgen-Nativbilder (in press).
7. Mundinger, F. (1975), Stereotaktische Operationen am Gehirn. Stuttgart: Hippokrates-Verlag.
8. Mundinger, F., Reinke, M.-A., Hoefer, Th., Birg, W. (1975), Determination of intracerebral structures using osseous reference points for computer-aided stereotactic operations. Appl. Neurophysiol. *38*, 3—22.
9. Peluso, F., Gybel S. J. (1969), Computer calculation of two target trajectory with "centre of arc-target" stereotaxic equipment. Acta Neurochir. (Wien) *21*, 173—180.
10. Schaltenbrand, G., Bailey, P. (1959), Introduction to stereotaxis with an atlas of the human brain. Vol. 1. New York: Grune and Stratton.
11. Thompson, C. J., Bertrand, G. (1972), A computer programme to aid the neurosurgeon to locate probes used during stereotaxic surgery on deep cerebral structures. Comput. Progr. Biomed. *2*, 265—276.

Authors' address: Prof. Dr. F. Mundinger, Medical Director at the Department of Stereotactic Neurosurgery and Neuronuclear Medicine, Neurosurgical Hospital of the University, Hugstetter Straße 55, D-7800 Freiburg i. Br., Federal Republic of Germany.

Acta Neurochirurgica, Suppl. 24, 109—119 (1977)
© by Springer-Verlag 1977

National Center "Ramón y Cajal" and Autonomous Medical School,
Madrid, Spain

Electrophysiological Set-Up for Data Acquisition and Processing During Stereotaxic Surgery: Demonstration on Pulvinar Units

W. Buño, Jr., J. G. Martín-Rodríguez, E. García-Austt,
and S. Obrador

With 8 Figures

Microelectrode recordings during human stereotaxic surgery have become a very important aid to the neurosurgeon during target localization, allowing for the correction of individual anatomical variabilities. These recordings permit the study of the electrical activity of the different nuclei reached by the electrode in its way towards the selected target. Moreover, the availability of digital computers in the physiological laboratories has greatly complemented the analysis of neuronal activity by the introduction of new and very powerful statistical techniques. The knowledge of specific patterns of unitary activity within the thalamic nuclei may give additional information useful for the localization of the target.

The use of unit recordings during stereotaxic surgery has particular difficulties. Operating rooms are equipped with large quantities of electrical apparatus that provide possible sources of interference. The size and mobility of the equipment also plays an important role. A display of the recordings and audiomonitoring of the spike activity should be available to the surgeon while he is advancing the microelectrode. A series of stimulating devices must also be available, while in many cases a record of tremor and/or of voluntary movements is necessary. Flexibility of the equipment is important in order to obtain as much data as possible in a relatively short time.

The purpose of this paper is to present a technical approach to be used in the acquisition and processing of data. Results will be presented mainly on the unitary activity recorded from the nucleus pulvinaris thalami (Pu). This nucleus was selected because it is the most common thalamic structure run through by a microelectrode from a posterior approach during the performance of stereotaxic surgery.

Data Acquisition

Patients, requiring a lesion in the thalamic nuclei (Vop-Vim, CM-Pf, or Pu) were operated under local anesthesia without pre-medication. The Leksell stereotaxic equipment was used. Conray

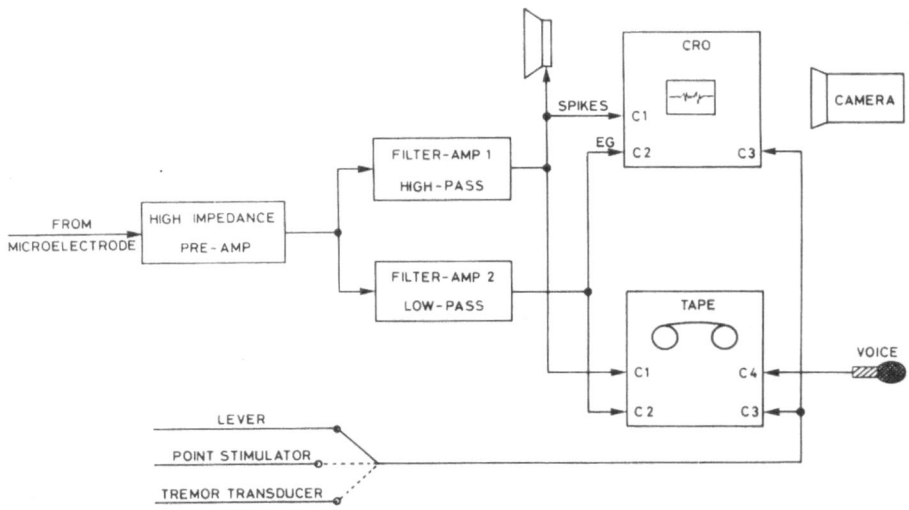

Fig. 1. Block diagram of data acquisition set-up (see text)

ventriculography was performed through a coronal burrhole. Target coordinates were referred to the AC-PC line and the midsagittal plane. In all patients microelectrode recordings of the thalamic nuclei were systematically obtained to aid correction of anatomical variability.

Extracellular unitary recordings were made with tungsten microelectrodes. Straightened tungsten wires of 0.5 mm diameter and 260 mm long were electrolytically etched (Hubel 1957) and insulated with varnish (Furniglass PU-15 Polyurethane Clear Varnish). Tungsten was selected as by far the stiffest, easily available metal. The microelectrode was placed in a protective cannula mounted on a carrier designed to fit the Leksell frame. The cannula was inserted through a posterior burrhole (in some cases from the coronal) and advanced with a micrometer drive attached to the carrier. Up to 30 mm could be explored in one track.

Fig. 1 shows the block diagram of the experimental set-up for data acquisition in the operating room. Voltages from the microelectrode were amplified with a high impedance preamplifier (Grass P 15) and simultaneously fed through two band-pass-filter amplifiers (Tektronix, mod. 26 A 2), one set as a high-pass and the other as low-pass-filter (cut-off 1–100 Hz and 0.1–10 kHz, respectively). With this procedure it is possible to separate unit and

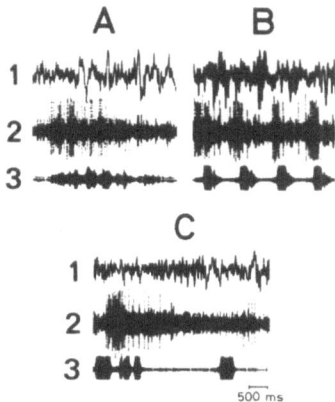

Fig. 2. Unit correlated with jaw movements. A) Recordings of gross activity (*1*) and unit activity (*2*) with the same microelectrode and separated by different band-pass filters, shown together with the patient's voice (*3*) as recorded from a microphone. In B) *1* and *2* same as in A) while (*3*) corresponds to the surgeon's voice indicating when the patient opens his mouth. C) *1* and *2* same as in A) and B), *3*, surgeon's voice ordering the patient to open (at the left of the record) and close his mouth (at the right)

gross activity obtained with the same microelectrode. In some cases, recordings of more than one constant amplitude spike with a good signal-to-noise ratio were obtained. Both activities were monitored in a CRO (Tektronix, model 5031 or 5103/D 13) and recorded separately on tape in a four-channel instrumental recorder (Hewlett-Packard, model 3960). Unit activity (spikes) was also monitored with a loudspeaker, providing immediate feed-back to the surgeon, allowing microelectrode positioning, and isolation of single units (Bates 1973). The third tape channel was used to record alternatively different electrical signals.

To have a time-reference of voluntary movements a specially designed pressing-handle was attached to the ipsi- or contralateral hand, from the recording site, providing a 1.25 V signal when pressed. A light emitting diode gave a visible indication of the performance. Skin tactile stimulation was made with a pin-point microswitch. The circuit provided a 1.25 V level when the skin was mechanically stimulated by a small lever attached to the switch. Changing the lever, a small or large area of skin could be stimulated (0.5 or 5 mm diameter). Tremor was recorded with a minute micro-

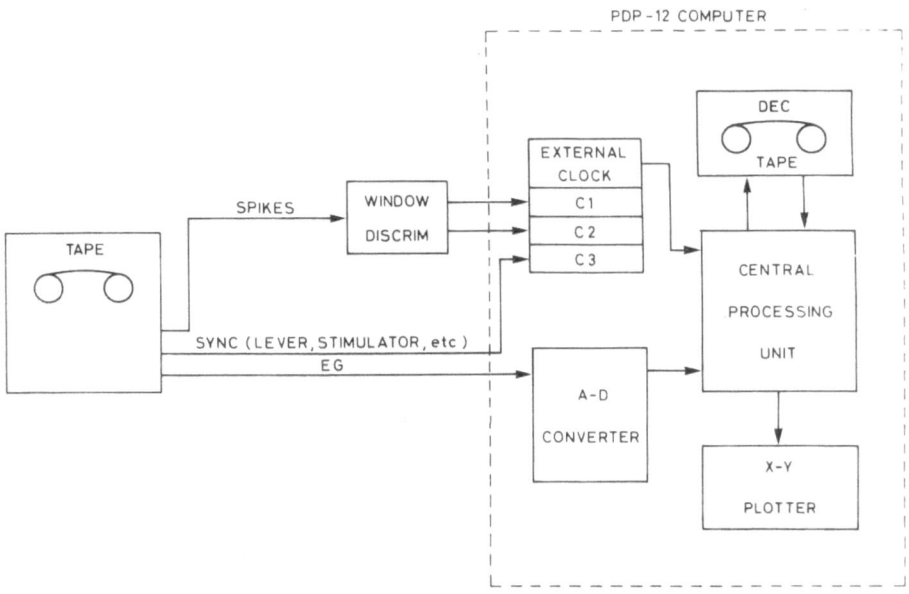

Fig. 3. Block diagram of data processing set-up (see text)

phone taped to the patient's hand. Its output was conveniently amplified and filtered. All these signals were monitored when necessary in the CRO.

Finally, electrode positions, patient performance, as well as any other interesting data, were verbally recorded in a voice-channel of the magnetic tape recording. Raw data could be on/or off-line photographed with a Polaroid model C-12 camera from the CRO storage screen.

In particular cases, one of the tape channels was used to record other timing signals. Fig. 2 shows a Pu unit that was correlated with jaw movements. In A through C, 1 represents the gross-activity and 2 the unitary activity recorded with the same microelectrode. A 3 is the recording of the patient's voice. The large spike (A 1) had a consistent time relationship with it. Further investigation of this unit indicated that it fired in relation with jaw movements. In B the patient was instructed to rhythmically open and close his mouth. B 3 is the recording of the surgeon's voice saying "open" every time the patient opened his mouth. A clear time relationship between the large unit and the patient's performance can be seen. In C he was instructed to maintain his mouth open. In C 3 at the beginning of the record, the surgeon ordered the patient to keep his mouth open.

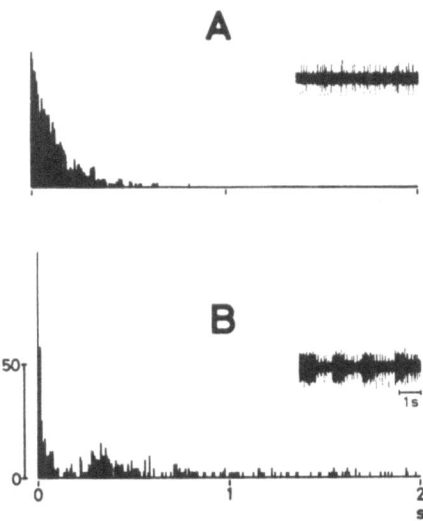

Fig. 4. Interspike interval distribution of two units firing spontaneously. A) Unit firing at random (insert) and interval histogram with a Poisson-like distribution. B) Unit firing in rhythmical bursts (insert) and histogram showing a bimodal distribution. A large initial peak, corresponding to intra-burst-intervals and small peak at 300 ms to inter-burst-intervals, can be seen

The unit fired with a burst decreasing in frequency and stopping even though his mouth was kept open. At the end of the record the patient was ordered to close his mounth and a smaller burst of spikes was elicited. The above findings indicate that this Pu unit shows a phasic relationship with jaw movements.

Data Processing

Thirty six Pu units were selected for processings. Data were processed off-line in a PDP-12 digital computer (16 K). Fig. 3 shows the diagram of the set up and of the connexions used for data processing. The components of the computer are represented inside the block limited by the broken lines. Tapes were played back with a tape recorder similar to the one used for data acquisition. Unit activity (spikes) was discriminated by amplitude and converted into pulses by a window discriminator (Frederick Haer mod. 40-75-1). One or two spikes could be processed simultaneously with the programes.

The programes * processed data in two successive stages. The first stage consisted in digitizing the data. The gross activity (EG) was sampled at a constant frequency in one channel of the computer's analog to digital converter. Intervals between pulses corresponding to spikes were also digitized in two channels of the external clock

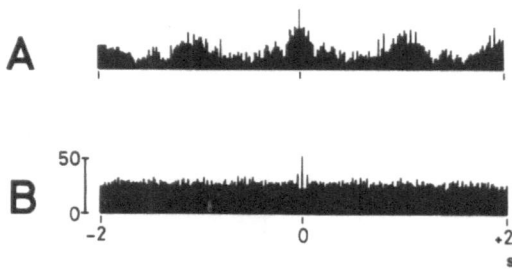

Fig. 5. Autocorrelation of the spontaneous firing patterns of two units. A) Unit firing with rhythmical bursts, as indicated by periodic peaks on either side of zero time. B) Unit firing at random, as shown by flat histogram indicating that the unit fires without a preferred interval

(with a precision of 1 ms), thus permitting the analysis of one isolated unit or two recorded simultaneously. The third channel of the clock was used for the timing pulses (sync). All these data were either stored in digital tape (DEC tape) or immediately processed. The resulting computed outputs were stored on DEC tape and plotted in the X-Y plotter (Hewlett-Packard model 7034 A).

Fig. 4 shows the distribution of the interspike intervals of two different Pu units firing "spontaneously". The length of the intervals are represented in abscissae and the number of interval occurrences in ordinates. Histogram A shows a Poisson-like distribution demonstrating a great number of short intervals with an exponential-like decay towards longer intervals. Histogram B indicates a bimodal distribution with a predominance of two different groups of intervals, the largest corresponding to shorter intervals. Inserts cor-

* The following programs were used: Promedio-Prom 200, P. Handler and N. Konickeski; Proceso, P. Handler, R. Budelli, O. Macadar (modified by J. Fuentes); Interv, J. Fuentes. Laboratory of Bioelectronics, Facultad de Medicina y Facultad de Ingeniería, Montevideo, Uruguay, and Department of Physiology, Autonomous University, Madrid, Spain.

respond to the raw unit recordings as photographed from the CRO screen. The data corresponding to histogram A, as indicated by its Poisson distribution, demonstrates that the unit is firing at random, a pattern which is not always apparent in the raw records. The distribution of intervals in histogram B is in acordance with the visual inspection of the raw data, showing rhythmical bursts. In some cases however, bimodal distributions do not correspond to rhythmic bursting activity. Furthermore, in particular cases, bursting activity may not have a bimodal distribution of intervals. This latter case

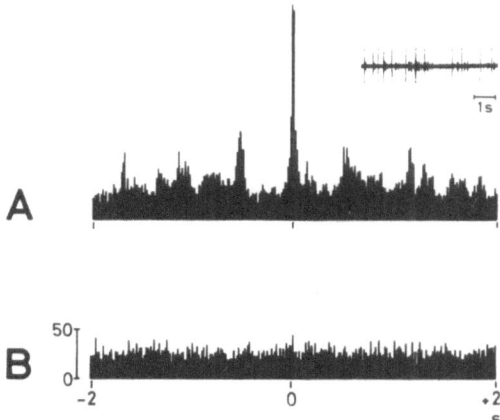

Fig. 6. Crosscorrelation of the spontaneous firing patterns of one pair of units. A) The firings of both units are correlated in time, the large unit (insert) was used as time reference (zero), the small unit fires in rhythmical burst in relation with the large spike as indicated by periodic peaks. Units recorded simultaneously with one microelectrode. B) Negative correlation of two units recorded simultaneously with the same microelectrode. Flat histogram indicating no preferred firing interval between the firings of both units

can be due to random bursting activity or to rhythmic activity with overlaying inter- and intra-burst intervals. More complex statistical measurements, *e.g.*, autocorrelations, which consider first order intervals and intervals of other higher orders may be necessary to show more complex firing patterns (see below).

Interval histograms which show the distribution of first order intervals are a simple statistical estimation giving a first approximation of the unit firing patterns. By comparing histograms of the same unit in different conditions they may also indicate changes in its firings. Moreover, Fig. 5 shows the two types of "spontaneous" firing patterns that are generally found in Pu units. Fig. 5 shows the auto-correlations of two different Pu units. A, corresponds to a unit firing

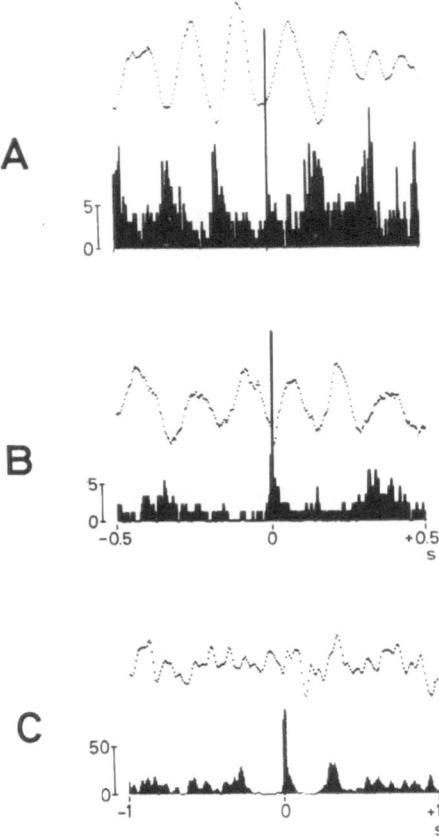

Fig. 7. Average of gross activity and firing probability of 3 different units made by synchronizing with spikes (zero time) (see text). A) and B) units firing in rhythmical bursts (lower record) in-phase with Pu rhythmical gross activity (upper record). The bursting activity of the unit in A has the same frequency of the gross activity rhythm, while the bursts in B) have one-half. C) Shows a unit that fires in random bursts and has no significant relationship with the gross activity. Averages of 50 epochs in A) and B), and 100 in C)

in rhythmical bursts. In abscissae, zero time corresponds to the firing of the unit. An epoch of 1 second before and 1 second after the firing was considered. Ordinates indicate the number of events corresponding to each bin or time division. The total number of spikes used to make this histogram was 730. This histogram gives an estimation of the firing probability of the unit an epoch before and after it fires. Periodic oscillations of the unit's probability of firing with an interval close to 0.5 s can be seen. B, is the autocorrelogram of a unit that fires at random. The histogram shows a constant amplitude demonstrating that there is no preferred firing interval. Autocorrelation functions are symmetrical if the amount of data used for their calculations is large enough and stationary. Again, both correlograms represent the two different types of units that were usually found in the pulvinar.

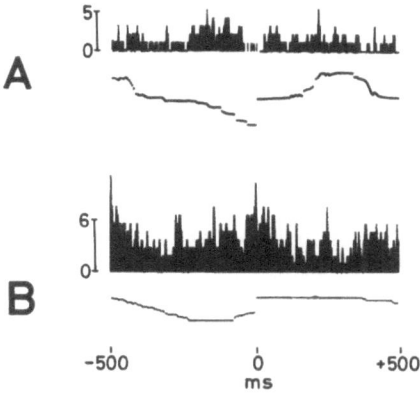

Fig. 8. Firing pattern of movement related Pu units in two different patients. A) and B) The upper histograms show the probability of firing of the units in relation with handle pressings (zero time). The lower records correspond to the averages of the voltage signal generated by handle pressings. In both cases results are the average of 50 successive epochs. (See text)

In cross-correlations between unit firings, zero time corresponds to the firing of one of the two units recorded with the same microelectrode, while the histogram shows the probability of firing of the other unit before and after zero time. Fig. 6 demonstrates the cross-correlation of two pairs of Pu units, A and B. The insert in A shows two units recorded with the same microelectrode. They were discriminated by amplitudes with the window discriminator. The firings of the large unit were used as zero time. The firings of both units were correlated in time, the small unit firing in rhythmical burst time-locked with the firings of the large one (see peaks at constant intervals). B, is an example of two other Pu units that show no timed relationship between spikes. This flat histogram indicates that units that are very close together (recorded with the same microelectrode) may not be related. Cross-correlation functions are usually asymmetrical.

The relationship between unit firings and gross activity was studied using an averaging method. Fig. 7 shows the histograms of the firing probability of three different Pu units. These histograms were made by synchronizing the averaging program with the spike (zero time) and considering the firing probability of the unit before and after the synchronizing action potential. This method is similar to the autocorrelation, but not all the intervals between spikes are considered because the program is only synchronized by spikes that are separated more than the interval corresponding to the analysis epoch. The upper record is the average of the gross activity synchronized with the same action potentials (similar to cross-correlation with spikes). In A and B, the averages of gross activity show rhythmical oscillations related in time with the spike firings, and the spikes also show rhythmical bursting activity. In A, both gross and unit rhythmical activity show the same frequency, while in B the unit fires once every two cycles of the gross activity. In C, no rhythmical activity can be observed; the unit had a tendency to fire in random bursts, as indicated by the central peak of the histogram surrounded by a region of low probability that is in turn surrounded by two smaller peaks. Two types of units have been found in the Pu, related and unrelated with the rhythmical gross activity.

The possible relationship between unit activity and rhythmical voluntary movements of the hand was also studied with an averaging program. In Fig. 8, A and B, the upper records show the histogram of the probability of firing of two different Pu units. The lower records correspond to the average of the voltage signal generated by the handle when pressed and released. Both graphs were constructed by synchronizing the averaging program with the signal corresponding to the pressing of the handle. In A, an increase of the firing frequency is observed immediately before the signal corresponding to pressings. In B, an increase of the firing probability follows the initiation of the handle pressing, and another smaller peak, probably in relation to the lever release, can be seen 300 ms before and after the zero time.

Conclusions

The study of the "spontaneous" activity of Pu has demonstrated that there are two main types of units. 1. Units firing in rhythmical bursts with frequencies ranging between 3 to 7 Hz, some of them phase-locked with the gross rhythmical activity having the same, or half of its frequency. 2. Units firing at random or in non-rhythmical bursts. These units did not show a significant relationship with the gross activity.

About 20% of the units studied showed a phasic relationship with voluntary movements. Limb movements and specially movements of the hands were studied. A small proportion of the units were also related to movements of the face and mouth. These patterns of activity can only be detected when using statistical methods such as those described above. The possible role of the Pu in motor activity, is suggested by the existance of movement related cells.

Acknowledgement

We acknowledge Dr. J.M.R. Delgado for his valuable support and advise.

References

Bates, J. A. V. (1973), Electrical recording from the thalamus in human subjects. In: Handbook of Sensory Physiology (Igo, A., ed.). Berlin-Heidelberg-New York: Springer.

Hubel, D. G. (1957), Tungsten microelectrodes for recording from single units. Science 125, 549—550.

Address for reprints: Dr. J. G. Martín-Rodríguez, Fresnedilla 2, Madrid-35, Spain.

Acta Neurochirurgica, Suppl. 24, 121–136 (1977)
© by Springer-Verlag 1977

Neurological Clinic for Nervous Disease and Stereotaxy Nakameguro,
Meguro, Tokyo, Japan

Estimation of the Neural Noise Within
the Human Thalamus

A. Fukamachi, Ch. Ohye, Y. Saito, and H. Narabayashi

With 10 Figures

Summary

We systematically studied neural noise patterns in 18 Parkinsonian patients
with the aid of an amplitude averaging circuit for quantitative estimation of the
neural noise level. In our anterolateral to posteromedial tracks, the following
results were obtained and discussed from practical points of view.

1. It is demonstrated that the variation of the neural noise level along the
descent of the electrode corresponds well to different subcortical structures, and
is therefore reliable for identifying them precisely.

2. In and around the VL nucleus, there were some differences in the neural
noise pattern between the medial and lateral groups. In the medial group (4 cases),
upper borders of the thalamus were clearly delineated, but lower borders were
not. Steep increases of the noise level were found about + 10 mm above IC-line
probably corresponding to the entrance of VL nucleus and the upper half of the
VL showed the highest level. On the other hand, in the lateral group (6 cases),
intrathalamic noise patterns were not so characteristic as medial group and noise
levels were lower. In three cases upper borders of the thalamus were not so
distinct. Lower borders were, on the contrary, more clearly distinguished than
the medial group.

3. Cases with simultaneous recordings with two electrodes in parallel with
frontal section were reported. This method was proved to be useful in delineating
the lateral edge of the thalamus, especially in the case with dilatation of the
third ventricle.

4. In the Vim nucleus, high levels of the neural noise were demonstrated.
Activity of kinesthetic neurons were mostly found, if any, among the higher noise
levels.

Introduction

In stereotactic operations for such extrapyramidal manifestations
as tremor, rigidity and athetosis, neurophysiological techniques as
well as radiological measurement are now essential for the precise
localization of the electrode tip in the depth of brain. For example,
observation of the single or multiple unit discharge with a micro-

electrode technique has been proved to be useful in delineation of the thalamic nuclei (Albe-Fessard *et al.* 1963, Jasper and Bertrand 1966, Velasco and Molina-Negro 1973).

Using the unitary recording technique we have already reported some functional aspects of the thalamus such as activity of sensory neurons and spontaneous burst discharges (Ohye *et al.* 1972, Ohye *et al.* 1974) and their practical aspect in relation to placing therapeutic lesion (Fukamachi *et al.* 1973). From these experiences, we have noted that different sites in the brain, or even in the thalamus,

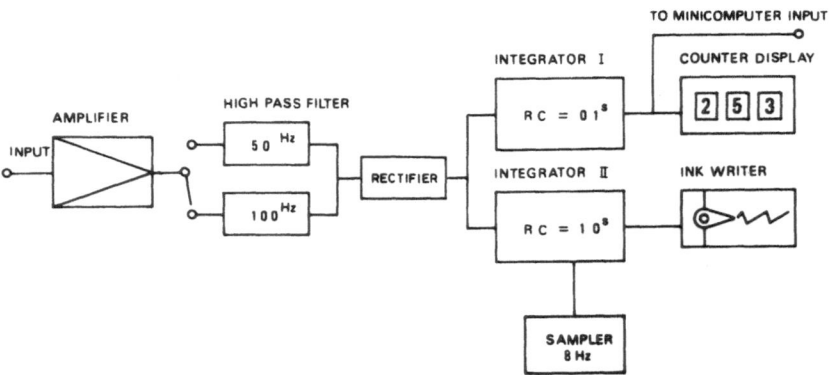

Fig. 1. Block diagram of neural noise quantification method or amplitude averaging circuit. 100 Hz—High Pass Filter is usually used. Explanation in the text

have different amplitudes of the neural noise. Here, the background neural noise is defined as a fast activity behind unitary spikes and such activity is believed to be over-all action potentials generated by cells and fibers surrounding the recording electrode. It is, therefore, conceivable that any difference in the amplitude of the neural noise denotes some anatomical difference.

Saito and Ohye (1974) developed an automatic or semiautomatic analog control device for micromanipulator motordrive. With a digital voltmeter in this system, quantitative estimation of level of the neural noise is always possible at each position during the course of insertion of the electrode. Neural noise levels thus obtained were proved to be very useful in delineating the thalamic nuclei and surrounding structure. We always use this quantitative estimation of the neural noise in addition to other electrophysiological devices for the precision in locating the target. In this paper we describe the neural noise quantification technique and a systematic study of the neural noise patterns within the human thalamus.

Materials and Methods

The present report is based upon observations made during stereotactic operations in 18 cases with Parkinson's disease. They were operated awake under local anesthesia with premedication of 10 mg of chlorpromazine. Operative targets were the ventralis lateralis (VL), ventralis intermedius (Vim) nuclei or sub-VL, Vim areas.

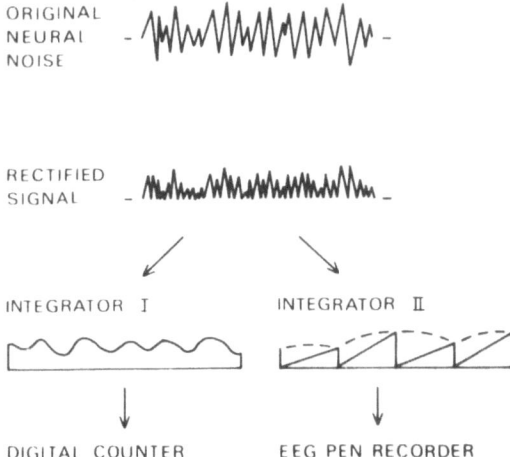

Fig. 2. Schematic figure for measurement of the neural noise level

The principal methods of the extracellular recording in the depth of brain were almost the same as those described in our previous papers (Ohye *et al.* 1972, Ohye and Narabayashi 1972, Fukamachi *et al.* 1973, Ohye *et al.* 1974). Briefly, an Insl-X coated bipolar concentric steel electrode (outer diameter: 0.6 mm, tip: 10–20 µm, resistance: 50–60 kΩ, distance between two poles: 0.5–1 mm) was introduced in an anterolateral to posteromedial direction through a frontal burr hole. As an analog control device was prepared for micromanipulator motordrive (Saito and Ohye 1974), the electrode was advanced at first by a rough manipulator in millimeter step and secondly, in the thalamus, especially in the ventral part, by an automatic micromanipulator in micron step. Bipolar recording between the two poles was usually made. In the majority only one needle track was used in each case. In two cases simultaneous recordings were made with two electrodes in parallel with frontal section, using a millimeter step manipulation. Frontal, pre- and post-central and occipital scalp EEGs were recorded throughout the whole operative procedure to monitor the patient's general cerebral activity. Surface bipolar electromyogram of the contralateral limb was also recorded on the cathode ray oscilloscope or pen-writing oscillograph. When sensory responses were obtained, touch, pressure or joint movement were signalled with a small strain gauge attached to the appropriate area.

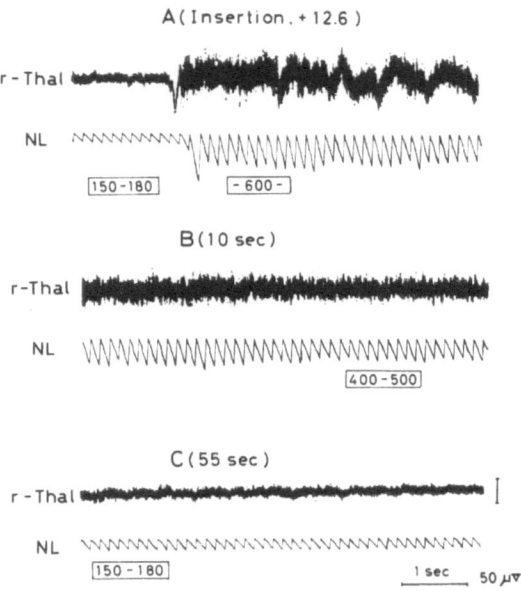

Fig. 3. An example of time sequential changes of transient mechanical injury discharge due to insertion of the electrode. Recording point is 12.6 mm above IC-line. A) Just at the insertion. B) 10 seconds after. C) 55 seconds after. Saw-tooth waves and numbers in squares indicate averaged neural noise levels. *Thal* thalamus, *NL* neural noise level

Recording and Measurement of the Neural Noise

In the case of deep-brain recording, suitably amplified with a high-gain amplifier, the neural activity was displayed on a cathode ray oscilloscope and photographed on a running film. If necessary, it was recorded on a jet-writer (Mingograf) during the course of insertion of the electrode. At the same time, it was also recorded on FM magnetic tape for later analysis and monitored on a loud speaker for facilitating the procedure.

Measurement of level of the neural noise was made through an averaging circuit as shown in Fig. 1. Output from the amplifier was led to a highpass filter with cut-off frequencies of 50 and 100 Hz. This filter was used to eliminate slow wave activity and pass only spikes to the next stage. These spikes were then rectified by a full-wave rectifier and the amplitude of rectified activity was half of the original neural noise. Rectified signal was further introduced

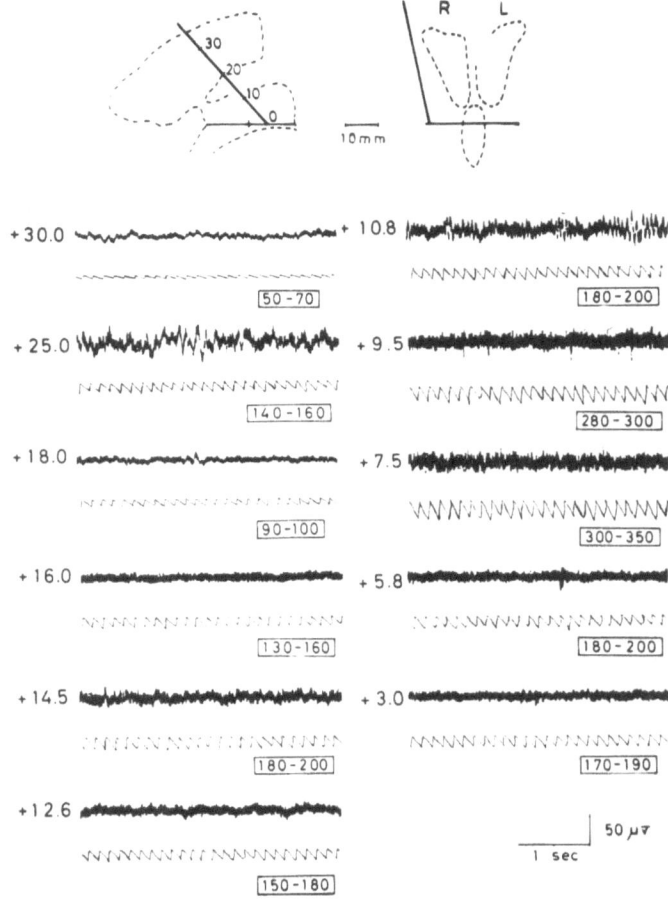

Fig. 4. Demonstration of recording and measurement of the neural noise in various depth of the brain in a 59-year-old woman with Parkinson's disease. Numbers indicate the distance in millimeters from IC-line. Upper two figures show the direction of the track projected to the shadow of the third ventricle in its lateral (left) and anteroposterior (right) views after pneumoventriculography. The intercommissural distance was 26 mm and the maximum width of the third ventricle was 6 mm as measured on X-ray. Saw-tooth waves and numbers in squares indicate averaged neural noise levels

into two kinds of integrator. Through integrator I with a short time constant (RC = 0.1 second), level of averaged amplitude of the neural noise was continuously displayed by a digital voltmeter. The number of two or three figures displayed on the counter indicates the value of about five times ($\times$ 10^{-}$^{-}$2) of averaged original noise amplitude in microvolts. When 253 is read as a level of neural noise, it denotes about 50 µV as an averaged amplitude of the original

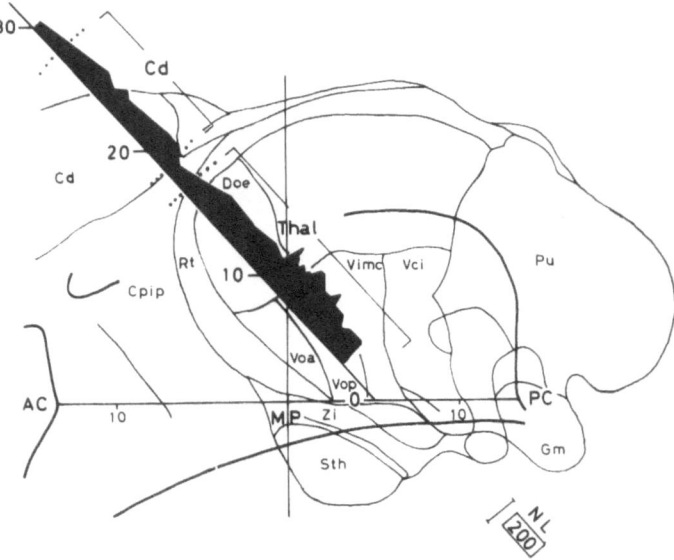

Fig. 5. Neural noise pattern of the case in Fig. 4 with a reproduction from Schaltenbrand and Bailey's atlas (S. 1. 13.5) and a lateral view of the third ventricle. Dotted lines indicate borders of the caudate nucleus (*Cd*) and thalamus (*Thal*). *AC* anterior commissure, *PC* posterior commissure, *MP* midpoint of IC-line, *NL* neural noise level

noise. On the other hand, through integrator II with a longer time constant (RC = 1 second) combined with 8 Hz-sampler, the averaged level of the neural noise was converted to amplitude of saw-tooth wave (8 Hz) and recorded on EEG pen recorder or jet-writer. Thus the level of the neural noise could be continuously read in two ways during the course of insertion of the recording needle. Fig. 2 shows a schematic drawing of the conversion mentioned above.

In general, at the time of insertion of the needle, the initial increase of the noise level due to so-called injury discharges was found (Fig. 3 A) and the level decreased gradually with the lapse of time (Fig. 3 B). In the present analysis of thalamic neural noise, the noise level at a given point was indicated by the stable level some time (20 to 60 seconds) after the insertion. In this illustrated case the noise level at this point was regarded as 150 to 180 (Fig. 3 C).

Although unitary large spikes distinguished from the background noise were also calculated in this system, their spontaneous discharge

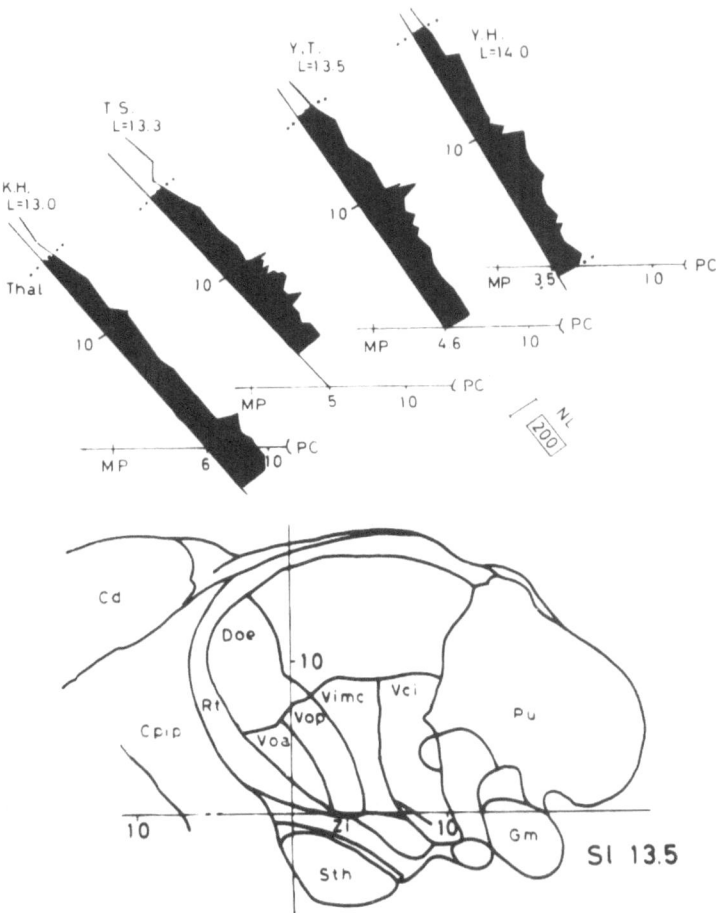

Fig. 6. Neural noise patterns in the medial group (4 cases) with a reproduction from Schaltenbrand and Bailey's atlas (S. 1. 13.5). "L = 13.0" indicates 13.0 mm lateral from midline on the level of IC-line. Dotted lines: borders of the thalamus (*Thal*). *MP* midpoint of IC-line, *PC* posterior commissure, *NL* neural noise level, numbers in millimeters

frequency was small in comparison with that of the background fast activity. The effect of unitary spikes to the noise level was therefore negligible.

Results

Case Presentation

A typical example of recording and measurement of the neural noise is shown in Fig. 4. This case was a 59-year-old woman with Parkinson's disease. Recording was made along a track penetrating toward the spot 5 mm behind the midpoint of intercommissural line (IC-line) and 13.3 mm lateral from the midline, as shown in the upper part of the figure.

In the white matter, or at a point + 30.0 mm above IC-line, level of the neural noise was 50 to 70 with frequent positive small spikes. In the caudate nucleus, or at a point + 25.0, it was around 150 with irregular wide spikes. At a point + 18.0, the level decreased again less than 100 suggesting that the needle had entered the white matter ventral to the caudate nucleus. When the tip of the electrode arrived at a point + 16.0, sudden increase of the noise level was found and this point was considered to be an upper limit of the thalamus. In the thalamus, various noise levels with some spikes or burst discharges were noticed at various points as shown in the figure. In the dorsal part of the thalamus levels of the neural noise were approximately 150 to 180. Upper half of the ventral part ($+ 9.5 \sim + 7.5$) revealed the highest level of the noise in the thalamus, the value being around 300. In the lower half of the ventral thalamus ($+ 5.8 \sim + 3.0$) a decrease of the level was found to be less than 200.

This continuous variation of the neural noise levels along its track was shown in Fig. 5, superimposed on a reproduction from Schaltenbrand and Bailey's atlas (S.1. 13.5) and a lateral view of the third ventricle. It was demonstrated that the neural noise variation corresponded well to subcortical structures and the caudate nucleus, white matter and thalamus were precisely delineated. Furthermore, in this case, ventral half of the thalamus corresponding approximately to the entrance of VL nucleus could be clearly distinguished from the dorsal one. Inferior limit of the thalamus could not be delineated in this case, because the recording needle was stopped at a point + 3.0 mm above IC-line.

As this demonstrats, variation of the neural noise levels gives us a continuous information along the descent of the electrode into subcortical structures, and therefore is reliable for identifying them precisely.

Different Noise Patterns Between Medial and Lateral Trackings

In the frontal view, tracks of recording electrodes penetrate through the subcortical structures between 13 and 18 mm lateral from midline on the level of IC-line. Difference of patterns of the thalamic neural noise levels within these limits was studied in 10 cases, especially with regard to medial and lateral tracks. Posterior limits of these cases were 1 to 6 mm behind the midpoint of IC-line and no responses were obtained to peripheral natural stimuli. These 10 cases were therefore considered to be concerned mainly with the VL nucleus. For the sake of convenience, tracks of 13 to 14 mm lateral from midline on the level of IC-line were grouped as medial and tracks of 15 to 16 mm as lateral.

Fig. 6 shows the neural noise patterns of the medial group (4 cases). As shown in the case presentation, changes of the intra-thalamic neural noise were characteristic. Steep rises of the noise level were found around a point $+ 10$ mm above IC-line and the levels of the upper half of the ventral thalamus were the highest in the thalamus. In the dorsal thalamus over $+ 10$ mm, levels of the neural noise were 150 to 180, in the ventral upper half 200 to 300 and in the ventral lower half less than 200. In the medial group, upper limits of the thalamus were usually clearly delineated, but lower limits were not so clearly demarcated. Only one in four cases showed a marked decrease of the noise level around IC-line.

Fig. 7 shows the noise patterns of the lateral group (6 cases). Although some degree of dispersion was seen, the noise levels of the lateral group were in general lower than those of the medial one. Rises of the noise levels around $+ 10$ mm above IC-line were not so marked as the medial group, but the higher levels were seen rather in the lower half of the ventral thalamus. Three cases (M. S., K. T., and F. I.) showed low levels of the neural noise with positive small spikes in the dorsal thalamus. In these three cases, upper limits of the thalamus were not so distinct. On the other hand, lower limits were more clearly distinguished in the lateral group than the medial one.

Fig. 8 shows two cases whose recordings were made simultaneously with two tracks in parallel with frontal section. Difference of the neural noise patterns between the medial and lateral tracks revealed the tendency described above. Especially in the case T. M., upper and lower limits of the caudate nucleus and thalamus were clearly demarcated. These simultaneous recordings revealed further the fact that the lateral and medial tracks had their respective upper and lower limits at different heights, being probably due to the anatomical shapes of the caudate nucleus and thalamus. From a practical point of view, it is important to evaluate the lateral edge of the thalamus when the dilatation of the ventricles, especially of the third ventricle, is found by radiological examination. In the case N. N., the third ventricle was 10 mm in width and dilated slightly. Neural noise levels on the lateral track penetrating a spot 18 mm

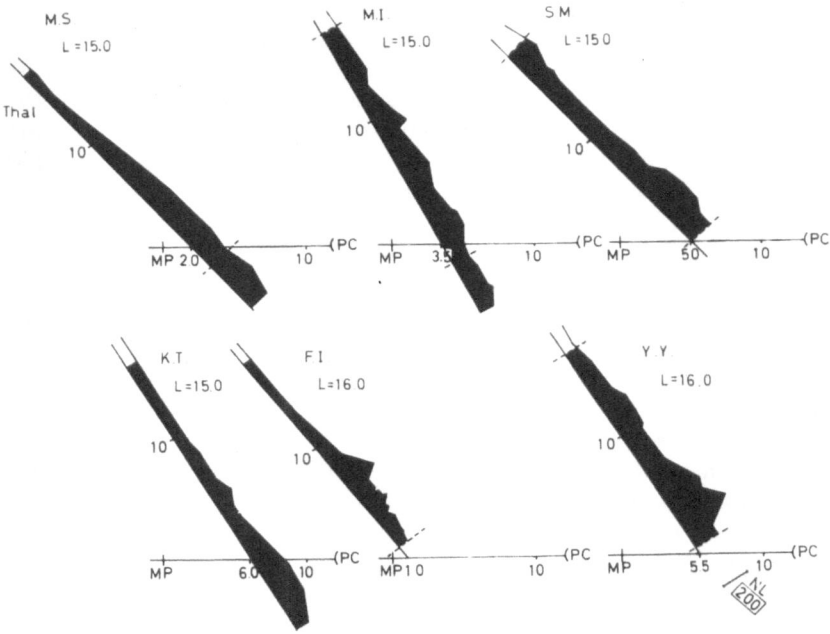

Fig. 7. Neural noise patterns in the lateral group (6 cases). Dotted lines indicate borders of the thalamus (*Thal*). *MP* midpoint of IC-line, *PC* posterior commissure, *NL* neural noise level, numbers in millimeters

lateral from midline were extremely low in comparison with the medial levels. The lateral track was therefore thought to pass through the very lateral part of the thalamus. On the other hand, in the case T. M., the lateral track penetrating a point 19 mm lateral from midline showed higher levels than the former case. It was accordingly conceivable that in the case with dilatation of the third ventricle there might be a reduction of the size of the thalamus itself.

Neural Noise Patterns in the Cases With Sensory Responses

In six cases, sensory neuronal responses to peripheral natural stimuli were obtained (Fig. 9). These tracks passed through posteriorly between 7.8 and 9.8 mm behind the midpoint of IC-line and laterally between 15.0 and 17.5 mm lateral from midline. Although sensory modalities were various (joint movement, passive stretch of muscle and deep pressure), purely tactile neurons were not encountered. These sensory neurons were therefore in a region between

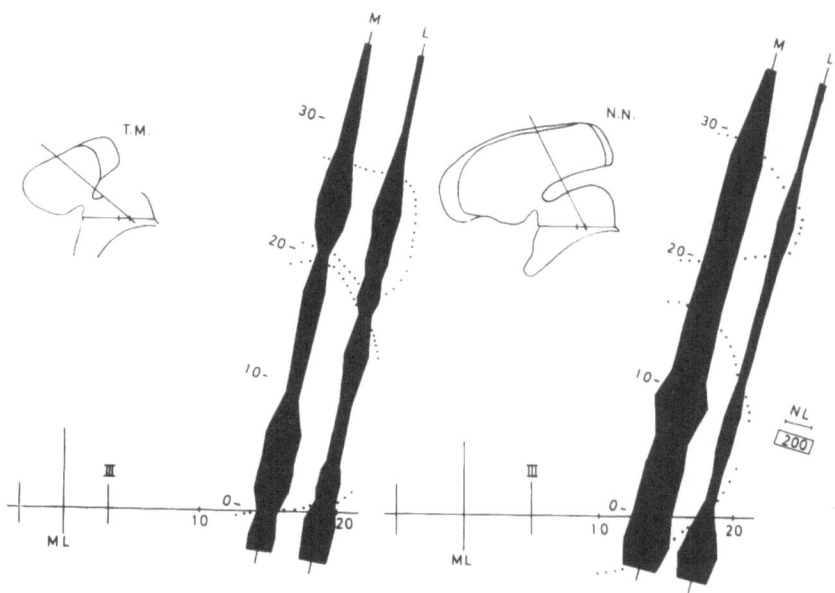

Fig. 8. An example of two cases with simultaneous recordings. In the case N.N. width of the third ventricle (III) was 10 mm and in the case T.M. 6.5 mm. Dotted lines indicate borders of the caudate and thalamus determined by changes of the neural noise. M medial track, L lateral track, ML midline, NL neural noise level, numbers in millimeters

the VL nucleus and the tactile area of the ventralis posterior. In one case (T. S.) evoked potential to peripheral nerve stimulation as that described by Goto et al. (1968) was obtained in this region. This region was thought to be the Vim nucleus.

Neural noise patterns in these cases were not so characteristic as the medial group mentioned above, but rather similar with the lateral group. Referring to the Schaltenbrand and Bailey's atlas, high levels of the noise were seen in the Vim nucleus. Kinesthetic neurons were mostly found among the higher background noise levels.

Difference of the noise level patterns between the VL and the Vim nucleus is not yet confirmed in individual case, but Figs. 6, 7, and 9 shows a tendency that the Vim nucleus has higher levels than the VL.

Finally one typical example of a 52-year-old male is presented in Fig. 10. Recording point is illustrated in B. Pressure on the left ankle evoked a multiunitary response in the thalamus. Neural noise was also elevated simultaneously. Digital voltmeter indicated around 300 before and over 400 just after the stimulation.

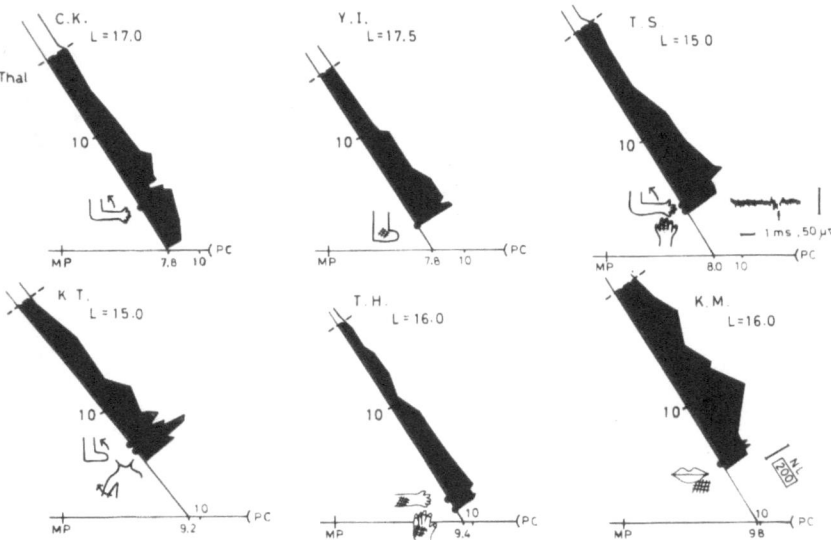

Fig. 9. Neural noise patterns in the cases with sensory responses (6 cases). Dotted lines indicate upper limits of the thalamus. Lower ones were not determined in these cases. Solid circles indicates the thalamic points of neurons with sensory responses. Schematic figures of a part of the body indicate the respective peripheral receptive field. The qualities of effective stimuli are indicated as follows: arrow; joint movement, a group of small dots; tapping, lattice; deep pressure. In the case T.S. an evoked response to median nerve stimulation is illustrated. *MP* midpoint of IC-line, *PC* posterior commissure, *NL* neural noise level

Discussion

Neural noise, or background fast activity, is thought to be primarily action potentials generated by cells and fibers surrounding the electrode (Arduini and Pinneo 1962, Podvoll and Goodman 1967, Schlag and Balvin 1963, Weber and Buchwald 1965, Buchwald and Grover 1970). It is also reported that the background activity is high in certain regions which are found to correspond to individualized nuclei or groups of nuclei (Schlag and Balvin 1963, Buchwald and

Grover 1970). Schlag and Balvin (1963) described that it was not yet possible to state whether size or density of cells or both, or additional factors were responsible for this result. Grover and Buchwald (1970), however, studied the correlation between the local morphology and the fast activity amplitudes. Their data suggested that neither fiber projections nor cell density contribute importantly to the differential large and small amplitudes of fast activity. They

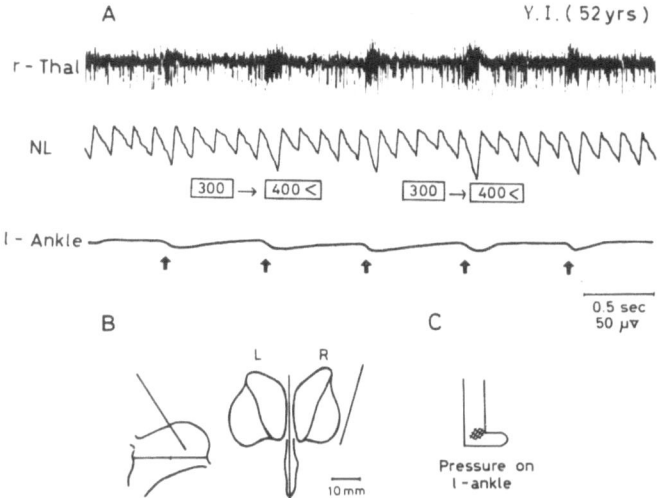

Fig. 10. An example of a case (Y.I. in Fig. 10) with sensory response. Deep pressure on left ankle was the effective stimulation (C in Figure). Thick arrows in A) indicate moments of the applied pressure. *Thal* thalamic recording, *NL* neural noise level. B) Recording point

concluded further that, in contrast, the fast activity amplitudes had shown a strong correlation with maximum cell diameter and seemed a more probable function of cell size than of the other variables. Therefore, it is conceivable that the background activity appears to be dependent upon the morphological characteristics of the cellular environment and the measurement of the activity level is valuable for localizing electrodes in the brain, as demonstrated in this paper.

Several investigators (Albe-Fessard *et al.* 1963, 1966, Hardy and Bertrand 1965, Hongell *et al.* 1973) described briefly the background activity in the human thalamus. However, there is no literature which concerned a detailed study on the neural noise patterns in the human thalamus, especially in the VL and Vim nuclei. Hongell *et al.* (1973) described that at a position 13 to 18 mm above IC-line there was an increase in spontaneous multiunit activity indicating the entry into the thalamus and at about 10 mm there was additional increase in overall activity probably indicating the entry into the VL nucleus. From our results, the medial group is similar to the description by Hongell et al., but the lateral one is not. In fact, the medial group revealed the higher levels in the upper half of the VL nucleus than the lower half. In the lateral group three cases showed a very low level with frequent positive small spikes in the dorsal thalamus. That is probably due to considerably lateral penetrations of needles or existence of more abundant myelin fibers in the dorsolateral region of the thalamus (cf., Dewulf's atlas, 1971). Accordingly when such low neural noise pattern is obtained, it must be considered that the electrode is penetrating through a fairly lateral part of the thalamus. In the thalamus, as far as examined by our anterolateral to posteromedial tracks, the Vim nucleus seemed to have the highest level of the neural noise. Cytometric studies by Dewulf et al. (1971), being the only available histological datum in the literatures, revealed that the Vim nucleus had larger macroneurons than the VL and the dorsal thalamus. This would be compatible with our results but further precise correlative study will be necessary.

In the case of the third ventricle dilatation, it is important to evaluate the size of the thalamus for determining an operative target. Assuming that atrophy of the basal ganglia can result in an increase of the width of the third ventricle (Selby 1968), placing a lesion in the same manner as in the persons with normal width may introduce such hazard as hemiparesis. Bogren et al. (1971) reported that the immediate result of the operation was better in patients with small than in those with wide third ventricles. As described in our results, assessment of the neural noise pattern is a good method for detecting the lateral border. Simultaneous recordings with two tracks in parallel with frontal section was proved to be more reliable in delineating the thalamus, especially its lateral edge.

Similarly the neural noise assessment was useful in distinguishing the upper and lower borders of the thalamus. Regarding the lower limit which is important for the sub-VL or sub-Vim thalamotomy, the lateral group demarcated it more clearly than the medial one, though the reason was not clear. Detail of this problem will be described separately elsewhere.

Finally, functional aspect will be discussed briefly. It is well known in animal experiments that there is a decline in the averaged multiple unit activity in the reticular and thalamic sites during the transition from wakefulness to slow-wave sleep (Podvoll and Goodman 1967, Goodman and Mann 1967). Although changes of the neural noise levels during wakefulness and sleep have not yet been reported in the human thalamus, it is likely that the similar phenomenon exists. In fact we have experienced several cases; in one case neural noise level was 180 to 200 while she was dozing, but it increased to 250 when she became more awake and tremor in the limb appeared. Neural noise patterns described in the results were therefore obtained in the stable states in regard to the patients' level of consciousness.

Acknowledgements

The authors are indebted to Prof. Jun-ichi Kawafuchi, Director of the Department of Neurosurgery, Gunma University, for his encouragement throughout this study.

They are also grateful to Mr. K. Ko, Misses M. Nagashima, M. Tateno, and K. Maegata for their technical and secretarial helps.

References

Albe-Fessard, D., Arfel, G., Guiot, G. (1963), Activités électriques caractéristiques de quelques structures cérébrales chez l'homme. Ann. Chir. *17*, 1185—1214.
— — — Derome, P., Hertzog, E., Vourc'h, G., Brown, H. Aleonard, P., De La Herren, J., Trigo, J. C. (1966), Electrophysiological studies of some deep cerebral structures in man. J. Neurol. Sci. *3*, 37—51.
Arduini, A., Pinneo, L. R. (1962), A method for the quantification of tonic activity in the nervous system. Arch. ital. Biol. *100*, 415—424.
Bogren, H., Wickbom, I., von Essen, C., Thulin, C. A. (1971), The width of the third ventricle in neurosurgical patients with extrapyramidal movement disorders. Confin. Neurol. (Basel) *33*, 120—128.
Buchwald, J. S., Grover, F. S. (1970), Amplitudes of background fast activity characteristic of specific brain sites. J. Neurophysiol. *33*, 148—159.
Dewulf, A. (1971), Anatomy of the normal human thalamus, Topometry and standardized nomenclature. Amsterdam-London-New York: Elsevier Publishing Company. 1971.
Fukamachi, A., Ohye, C., Narabayashi, H. (1973), Delineation of the thalamic nuclei with a microelectrode in stereotaxic surgery for parkinsonism and cerebral palsy. J. Neurosurg. *39*, 214—225.
Goodman, S. J., Mann, P. E. G. (1967), Reticular and thalamic multiple unit activity during wakefulness, sleep and anesthesia. Exp. Neurol. *19*, 11—24.
Goto, A., Kosaka, K., Kubota, K., Nakamura, R., Narabayashi, H. (1968), Thalamic potentials from muscle afferents in the human. Arch. Neurol. *19*, 302—309.
Grover, F. S., Buchwald, J. S. (1970), Correlation of cell size with amplitude of background fast activity in specific brain nuclei. J. Neurophysiol. *33*, 160—171.
Hongell, A., Wallin, G., Hagbarth, K. E. (1973), Unit activity connected with movement initiation and arousal situations recorded from the ventrolateral nucleus of the human thalamus. Acta Neurol. Scand. *49*, 681—698.
Jasper, H., Bertrand, G. (1966), Thalamic units involved in somatic sensation and voluntary and involuntary movements in man. In: The Thalamus, pp. 365—390 (Purpura, D. P., Yahr, M. D., eds.). New York: Columbia University Press.

Ohye, C., Fukamachi, A., Narabayashi, H. (1972), Spontaneous and evoked activity of sensory neurons and their organization in the human thalamus. Z. Neurol. *203*, 219—234.

— Narabayashi, H. (1972), Activity of thalamic neurons and their receptive fields in different functional states in man. In: Neurophysiology studied in man, pp. 78—89 (Somjen, G. G., ed.). Amsterdam: Excerpta Medica.

— Saito, Y., Fukamachi, A., Narabayashi, H. (1974), An analysis of the spontaneous rhythmic and non-rhythmic burst discharges in the human thalamus. J. Neurol. Sci. *22*, 245—259.

Podvoll, E. M., Goodman, S. J. (1967), Averaged neural electrical activity and arousal. Science *155*, 223—225.

Saito, Y., Ohye, C. (1974), Automatically controlled recording and processing of thalamic unit discharges in human stereotaxic operation. Confin. Neurol. (Basel) *36*, 314—325.

Selby, G. (1968), Cerebral atrophy in parkinsonism. J. Neurol. Sci. *6*, 517—559.

Schlag, J., Balvin, R. (1963), Background activity in the cerebral cortex and reticular formation in relation with the electroencephalogram. Exp. Neurol. *8*, 203—219.

Velasco, F., Molina-Negro, P. (1973), Elektrophysiological topography of the human diencephalon. J. Neurosurg. *38*, 204—214.

Weber, D. S., Buchwald, J. S. (1965), A technique for recording and integrating mutiple unit activity simultaneously with the EEG in chronic animals. Electroenceph. clin. Neurophysiol. *19*, 190—192.

Authors' addresses: Drs. A. Fukamachi and C. Ohye, Department of Neurosurgery School of Medicine, Gunma University, 3-39, Showa-Machi Maebashi, Gunma, Japan, and Dr. Y. Saito, Department of Neuropsychiatry, Faculty of Medicine, University of Tokyo, 7-3-1, Hongo, Bunkyo-ku, Tokyo, Japan.

Acta Neurochirurgica, Suppl. 24, 137—138 (1977)

Department of Neurosurgery, Beth Israel Hospital and Harvard Medical School

Technical Factors in Stereotaxic Hypophysectomy

N. T. Zervas and H. H. Hamlin

In previous reports to this society [1], we have described the results of radiofrequency thermal hypophysectomy in patients with metastatic breast and prostatic cancer and diabetic retinophaphy. At the present time, we are able to document panhypopituitarism in 91% of all patients. Using the experience gained with operations on over 400 patients, we should like to stress some of the technical factors which reduce complications.

Diabetes insipidus: this complication follows all operations if panhypopituitarism is achieved. However, 5% of all patients develop polyuria that requires therapy for more than three months. Therapy with chlorpropamide 250 mg (given daily is usually sufficient to control late problems with diabetes insipidus and only rarely is pitressin tannate injection necessary. This problem can probably be minimized, if attention is paid to limiting the size of lesions near the posterior superior surface of the gland. To do this, we do not produce thermal lesions (80 degrees Centigrade) for more than 30 seconds in this zone.

Visual complications: two patients suffered permanent bitemperal hemianopsia. In both instances, extension of the side arm of the thermal electrode above the sella turcica could be documented. The absence of the diaphragma sellae in these cases probably permitted the upward extension of the electrode tip. However, it would seem prudent to be certain that the electrode never approaches a line drawn from the dorsum sellae to the tuberculum sellae. In this way, direct contact of the electrode tip with a low lying optic chiasm will be avoided. In any case, the electrode should be monitored with plane X-ray films prior to each lesion to insure that the tip is within the sella turcica.

Cerebrospinal fluid rhinorrhea: in the past, 14 cases of rhinorrhea with seven instances of meningitis developed. In the past two years, these complications have not occurred. The tactic of packing the sella turcica with small squares (3 × 3 mm) of bovine fascia lata (Ethicon) to occlude the electrode tract appears to have been successful. In addition to this a malleable dumbbell shaped silicone plug impregnated with silver is forced into the bony hole in the anterior wall of the sella turcica. Both maneuvers apparently have led to the minimization of this serious complication. It is the authors' opinion that the packing of the sella with the fascia lata is the most important step necessary to prevent rhinorrhea.

We also explored the use of remote induction heating for hypophysectomy [2]. We concluded that the hazards of this technique, primarily, arcing of high voltage R F current from the induction coil to the patient's head was not yet overcome.

References

1. Zervas, N. T., Stereotaxic thermal hypophysectomy. Progr. neurol. Surg. 6, 21—25. Basel: Karger.
2. Zervas, N. T., Shintani, A., Kuwayama, A., Hale, R., Pickren, K. S., Merry, A., Experimental induction heating hypophysectomy. Confin. Neurol. (Basel) 35, 129.

Authors' address: N. T. Zervas, M.D., Department of Neurosurgery, Beth Israel Hospital and Harvard Medical School, 330 Brookline Avenue, Boston, MA 02215, U.S.A.

Acta Neurochirurgica, Suppl. 24, 139—147 (1977)

Institute of Neurology (Chairman: Prof. E. Csanda), Semmelweis Medical University, Budapest, Hungary

Structural, Ultrastructural and Functional Reactions of the Brain After Implanting Yttrium 90 Rods Used in Stereotactic Neurosurgery

E. Csanda, F. Joó, I. Somogyi, A. Szücs, M. Saal, A. Auguszt, and S. Komoly

With 10 Figures

Introduction

In stereotactic neurosurgery the implantation of beta irradiating Y 90 rods for producing circumscribed lesions in the brain has been successfully used for a long time, as for instance in the impressive series of frontal psychochirurgical lesions done by Dr. Knight. Dr. Talairach's team in Paris used the same type of radioactive lesionmaking. Whilst lesions in the gray matter appeared to be regular and satisfactory from the clinical and histological point of view, after more extensive lesions of the white matter of the hemispheres some side effects appeared, consisting mainly in more or less marked phenomena of brain oedema in about 20%. In 1970 with Szikla and Vedrenne [1, 2] we gave a first account of the histological alterations of the brain tissue provoked by focal irradiation. Later we extended these examinations on animal experiments and completed it with analysing the permeability changes [3, 4, 5].

Material and Methods

In our present work we give an account of 240 experiments carried out mainly on dogs and cats and in smaller number on rabbits and rats. Y rods of 0.10–2.4 mCi activity were implanted into the cortex, or stereotactically into the deep white matter and subcortical nuclei such as caudate and hippocampus. Neuropathological examinations were carried out from 4 hours to 16 months after implantation. Six cats were perfused with Karnovszky solution and examined electronmicroscopically.

To analyse macroscopically the BBB disturbances and the extent of the edematous reactions, 102 animals were given 25 mg/body weight kg Evans blue 24 hours before decapitation. EEG recordings were made in 12 animals.

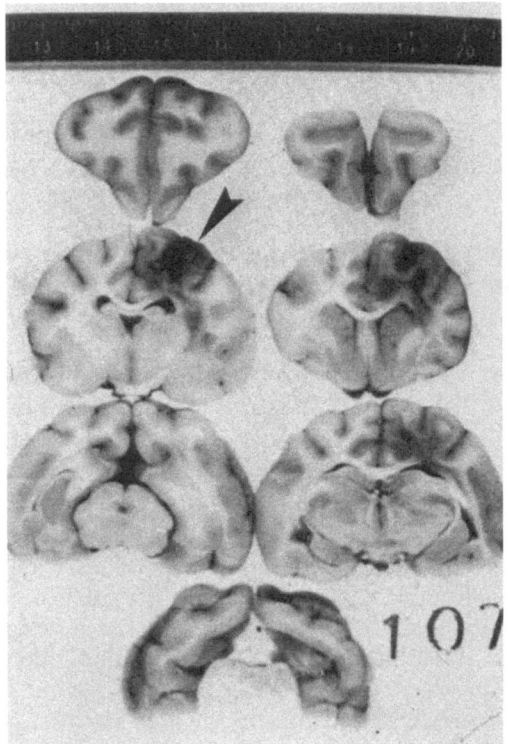

Fig. 1

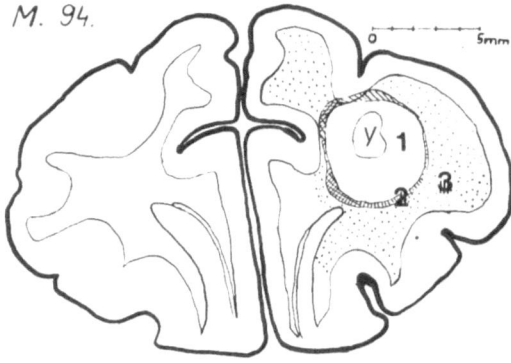

Fig. 2

Therapeutic experiments were performed to test three substances in preventing the perifocal oedema. One group of the animals was administered 2 gr/body weight kg glycerol three times daily, the second group received 0.5 mg Oradexon twice a day, and the third one was in every four hour given a solution of 0.2 mM Metiamid (0.5 ml/body weight kg). Metiamid—a new antihistaminic substance—acting on H_2 receptors is supposed to be an antiedematogenic. Dr. Joó.

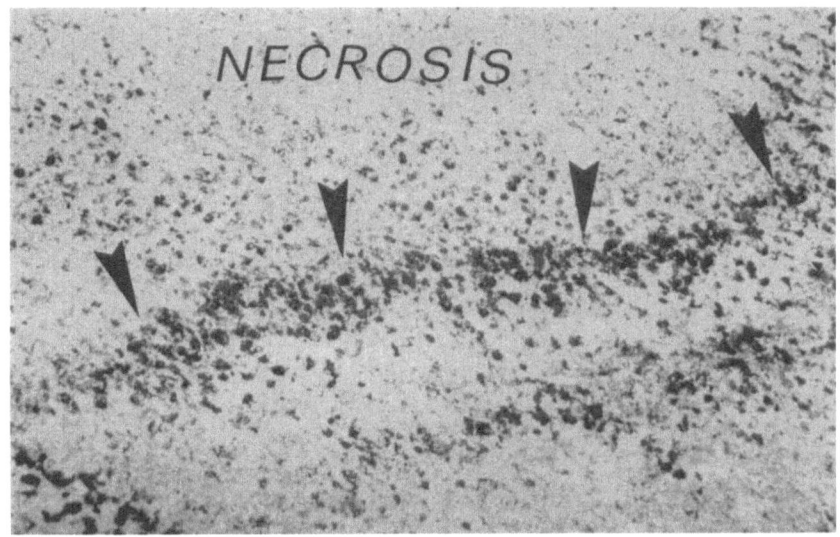

Fig. 3

Results

We restrict our results and report and demonstrate only those bearing some correlation with stereotaxy.

The cortical implantation results in a perifocal edema giving a light blue staining with Evans blue, while the perinecrotic area turns into dark blue on staining, as it can be seen on Fig. 1 representing a cat's brain three days after implanting a rod of 1 mCi. The edematous reaction is more marked when we implant the rod into the deep white matter. Whilst the size of the necrosis is essentially the same in every case, the degree and speed of the oedematous reaction depends on the activity of the rods and is the highest always on the third-fourth day.

The Evans blue method shows the protein content of the brain oedema in a semiquantitative way. The deeper the staining, the greater the protein content, as is proved with Masson and PAS

staining. Beside a diffuse PAS staining several PAS positive astro-
cytes can be found, the persistance of which depends on the activity
of the rods and the species of the animals.

Fig. 2 is a sketch of the histological alterations found in a cat's
brain after four days around a 1 mCi rod. The zone 1 represents

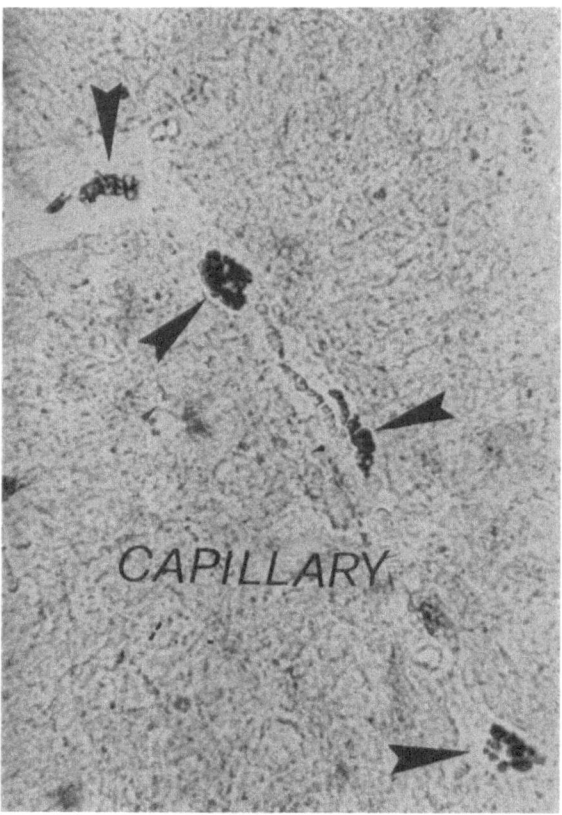

Fig. 4

the necrotic area, zone 3 the perifocal oedema discussed above. The
zone 2 being a narrow one, is very active. Besides a mesodermal
and glial proliferation there is seen to be a fluid accumulation as
well as a myelin damage. The fluid accumulated between the axon
and its myelin sheath and the mesaxon broken off from its envelope.
An other type of alteration is characterized by extremely enlarged
pseudo-extracellular spaces appearing as the consequence of mem-

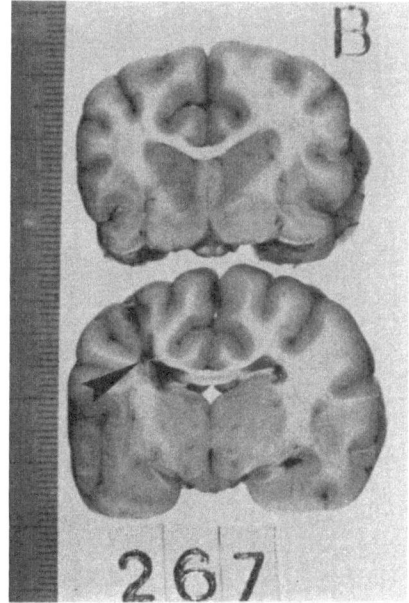

Fig. 5

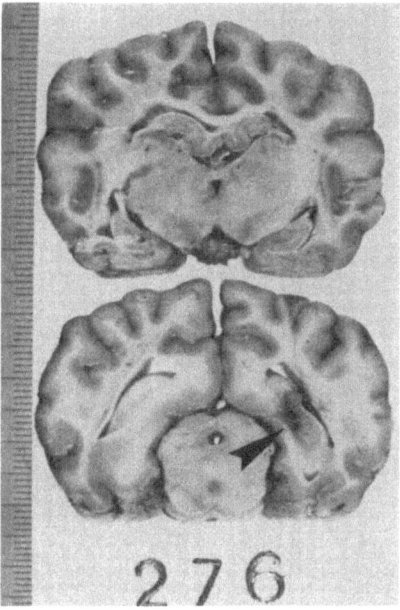

Fig. 6

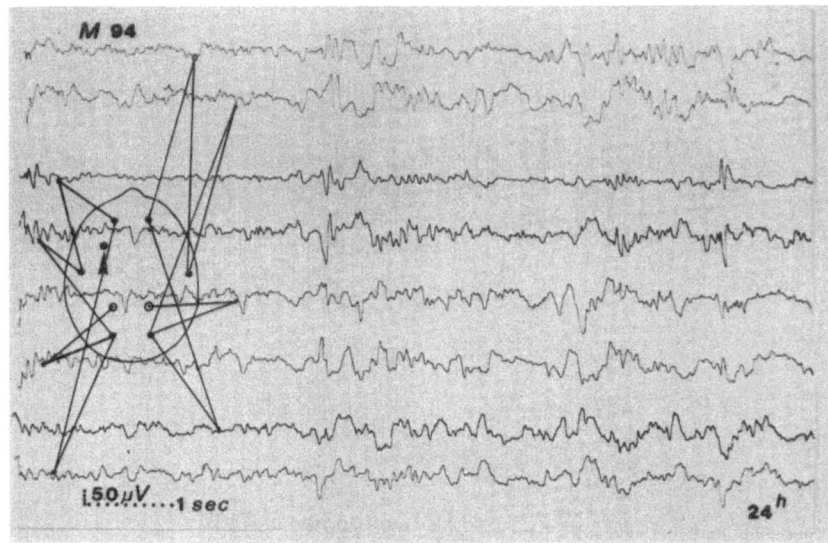

Fig. 7

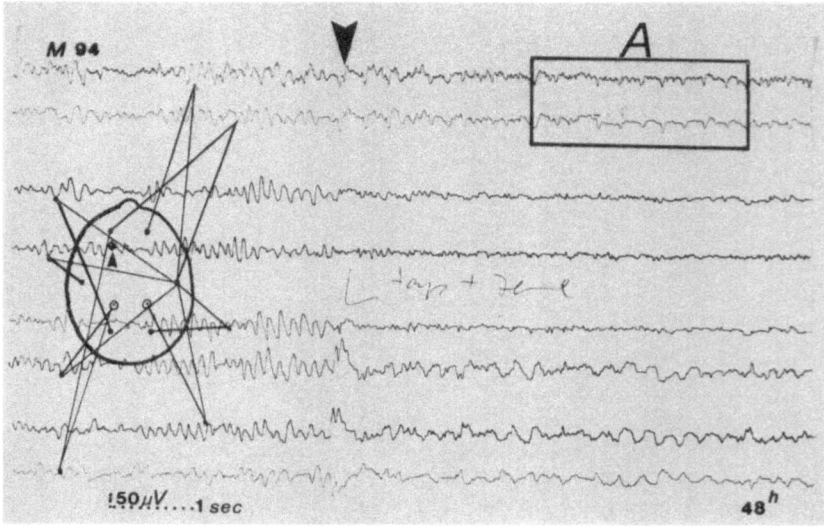

Fig. 8

brane damages. The myelin sheaths evaginated into these spaces in a peculiar way. In the same zone a large amount of Sudan positive decomposed substances can be detected (Fig. 3, see arrows). The cells containing Sudan positive substances migrate to the wall of the blood vessels, along which the transport of these substances can be observed (Fig. 4, see arrows). This process is going on even when

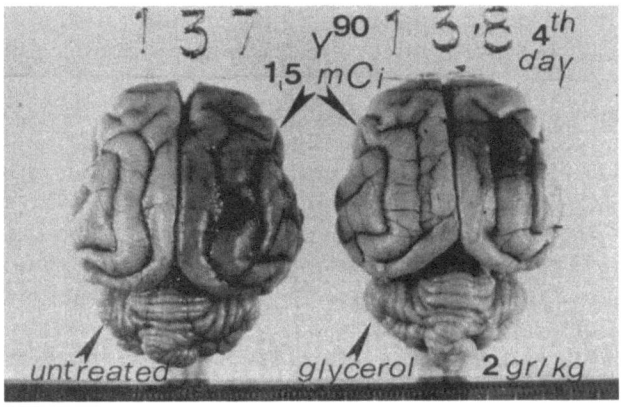

Fig. 9

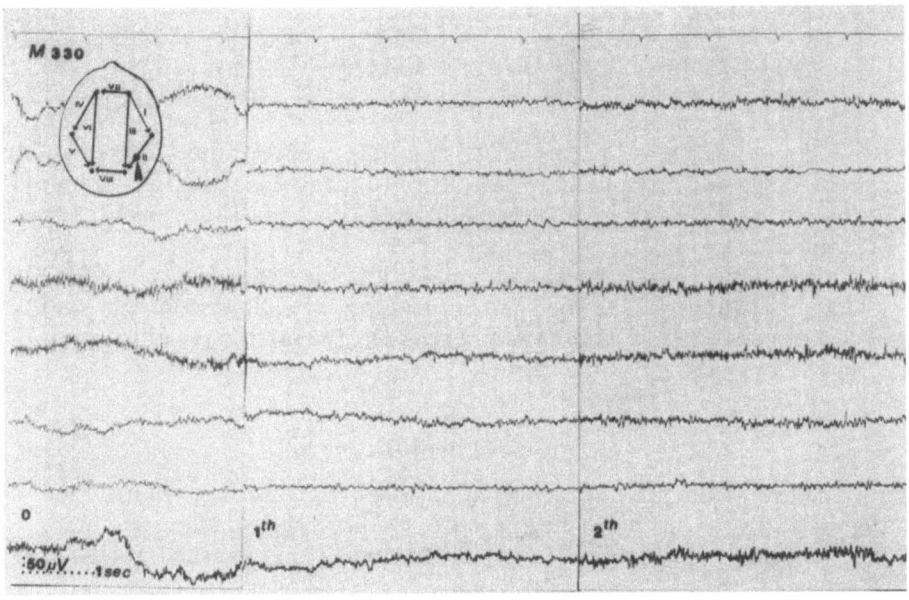

Fig. 10

the rods have long lost their activity. If the implantation was performed in the white matter, this progressive demyelinating process
can produce a marked decrease of the white matter as is demonstrated in Fig. 5 on the left side, representing a dog's brain ten
months after implantation of a rod of 0.5 mCi (the arrow indicates
the place of the rod). On Fig. 6 there is no difference in the white
matter of the two hemispheres, as the implantation (0.5 mCi) was
performed in the right hippocampus (nine months earlier).

It is to be noted, that no neurological signs or behaviour
disturbances could be observed in any of these animals. In general it
is only during the first week, following implantation, that the signs
of fatigue and anorexia can be observed if the rod has had high
activity level, or has been implanted in the deep white matter. We
have never seen any epileptic seizures.

EEG recordings made with epidural and deep electrodes show
remarkable alterations. Even after implanting the rod into the deep
white matter sharp waves appear beside the slow ones within
24 hours following implantation (Fig. 7). After 48 hours on clicking
or stimulating the animal in any other way, desynchronization sets
in, but on the side of implantation the beta activation fails to appear
(A on Fig. 8). In the deep electrodes the slow wave activity becomes
more pronounced. We tested antiedematous substances out of which
glycerol was more efficient than the steroids. Fig. 9 demonstrates two
dog brains three days after cortical implantation with the same high
activity, the animal on the right side was treated with glycerol.

Even a more striking effect can be observed in the case of
Metiamid treatment.

As contrasted with Figs. 7 and 8, representing the EEG
recordings of an untreated cat, Fig. 10 demonstrates, that under
the effect of Metiamid treatment the EEG does not show any significant alteration, even on the second day. It is only on the fourth
day, that the focal activity gets more pronounced, and only the fifth
day, that there appear the signs of a moderately slower activity and
sharp waves. The same effectiveness of the Metiamid therapy is
shown by the Evans blue method.

Conclusion

We should like to emphasize, that circumscribed destruction
practically of the same size can also be produced in the brain with
Y 90 rod of low activity, without inducing any marked perifocal
oedema.

The lesions caused by implanting the rod into the grey matter remain circumscribed, while the implantation performed in the white matter induces a slowly progressive demyelination, without damaging the cortex itself. This fact can be of some interest in psychosurgery.

References

1. Vedrenne, Cl., Csanda, E., Fontaine, Ch., Szikla, G. (1970), Analyse histologique des lésions précoces et tardives par l'implantation intracérébrale chez l'homme d'un isotope emetterur bete: l'yttrium 90. Comptes rendus du VIᵉ Congrés Internat. de Neuropathol, pp. 275—276. Paris: Masson.
2. Csanda, E., Szikla, G., Vedrenne, Cl. (1970), Étude expérimentale des modifications de la barrière hémo-encephalique sous l'effet du rayonnement beta. Comptes rendus du VIᵉ Congrés Internat. de Neuropathol., pp. 271—272. Paris: Masson.
3. Csanda, E., Szücs, A., Dobranovics, I. (1972), Tierexperimentelle Beiträge zu dem durch einen Beta-Strahler (Yttrium 90) verursachten Hirnödem. 2. Donausymposion für Neuropathologie. Wiener klin. Wschr. *84*, 435.
4. Csanda, E., Szücs, A., Dobranovics, I., Saal, M., Oswald, A. (1974), Hirnschädigungen infolge von Beta-Strahler Yttrium 90. Weitere Untersuchungen zur Frage der prälymphatisch-lymphatischen Drainagebahn aus der Hirnsubstanz. Folia Angiologica *22*, 172—174.
5. Csanda, E., Szücs, A., Joó, F., Dobranovics, I., Saal, M., Oswald, A. (1974), Experimental data to the alterations of the central nervous system following beta irradiation. Proc. of the VIIᵉ Internat. Congr. of Neuropathol. Budapest, 1974, pp. 765—768.

Authors' address: Dr. E. Csanda, Balassa utca 6, 1083 Budapest, Hungary.

Section III

Neurophysiology

Acta Neurochirurgica, Suppl. 24, 151—157 (1977)
© by Springer-Verlag 1977

National Institute of Neurosurgery, Budapest, Hungary

The Study of Recovery and Modification of the Evoked Potentials and Motor Answers in the Motor System

Sz. Tóth, J. Vajda, and P. Zaránd

With 4 Figures

Summary

After an electrical stimulus within the motor system there will follow a compulsion, a reflexlike process in functional dependency, naturally in illness (function disturbance) dependency as well. We can detect this process with the evoked potentials at the non-stimulated sites of the motor system and with the motor answers at the periphery. Because the motor system acts as a whole, it is certain that every process at a site has its correlates at the other sites, but the different part of the same process will be in a different grade pronounced (many times in opposite direction) at the different sites. If we want to know something from the basic process and to find the real correlates, we have to compare different evoked potentials within the motor system and motor responses at the periphery, or we have to enhance or depress the whole process or its parts. For the latter the double stimulation technique is suitable, but we have to take into consideration that during this investigation two alternating processes affect each other and therefore the result will not be direct.

From the time of Sherrington's investigation it is well known that behind the voluntary innervated "prime movers" work many voluntary evoked reflexes, automatic and semiautomatic movements. It means that within the motor system there never exists an isolated movement because it is a complicated process and the movement itself is only one item. The same is true for the reflex activity as verified by the H-reflex recovery investigation (Magladery and McDougall 1950, Paillard 1955). From our previous studies (Tóth 1972, Tóth, Zaránd, and Lázár 1974, Tóth and Zaránd 1972–1973) it is quite clear that a stimulus within the motor system is followed by a longlasting (300–1,000 ms or more) alternating facilitation and inhibition process. This process depends on the stimulus parameters, the site of stimulation and on the functional state of the motor system (Tóth, Zaránd, and Lázár 1974, Tóth, Zaránd, Lázár, and Vajda 1975). One could follow these changes from the evoked potentials at the non-stimulated sites of the motor system and from the evoked changes of the electrical activity of the muscles during

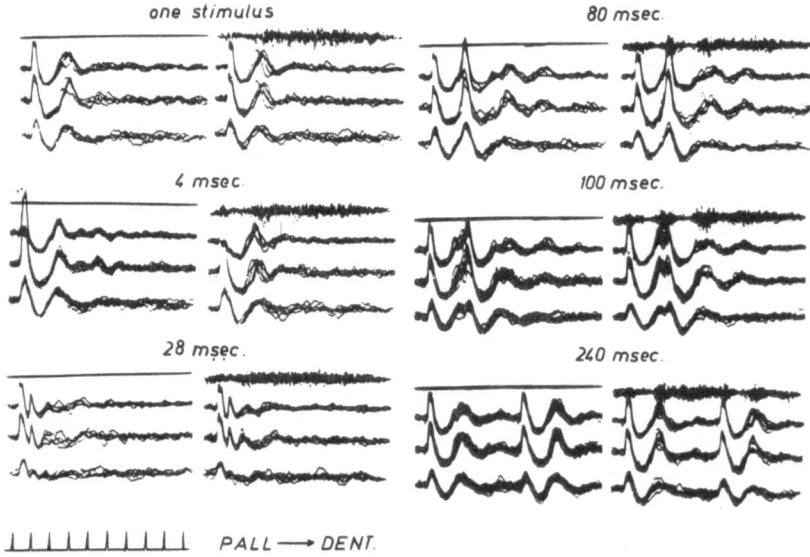

Fig. 1. Parkinsonism. Stimulation of the right pallidum with single and double stimuli (15 V, 0.05 msec). Registration from three different point of the brachium conjuctivum-dentate nucleus complex on the left side and from the left biceps muscle in rest and during voluntary contraction, with very little functional changes. Time calibration for all the figures 50 msec between two spikes. Calibration of the amplitude 0.05 mV in the EEG and 1 mV in the myogram

voluntary contraction. Usually between the different parts of the evoked potentials and the enhanced and depressed part of the electrical activity of the muscles there are quite strong correlations.

The main task of our recent investigation was to detect by the means of double stimuli how the second stimulus modifies the answer to the first and how the first stimulus modifies the answer to the second phenomenologically and from the point of view of facilitation and depression.

The investigations were made on patients with chronically implanted platinum or gold electrodes in the cases of epilepsy, central pain or movement disorders. In the last ten years we worked out the multitarget technique for the operation of movement disorder and central pain (Tóth 1972, Tóth, Zaránd, and Lázár 1974, Tóth and Zaránd 1972–73, Tóth, Zaránd, and Vajda 1976). This technique gives us the possibility to study the motor system including the ventrolateral nucleus of the thalamus, the pallidum, the dentate nucleus, the cerebellar cortex, the motor cortex, the centrum media-

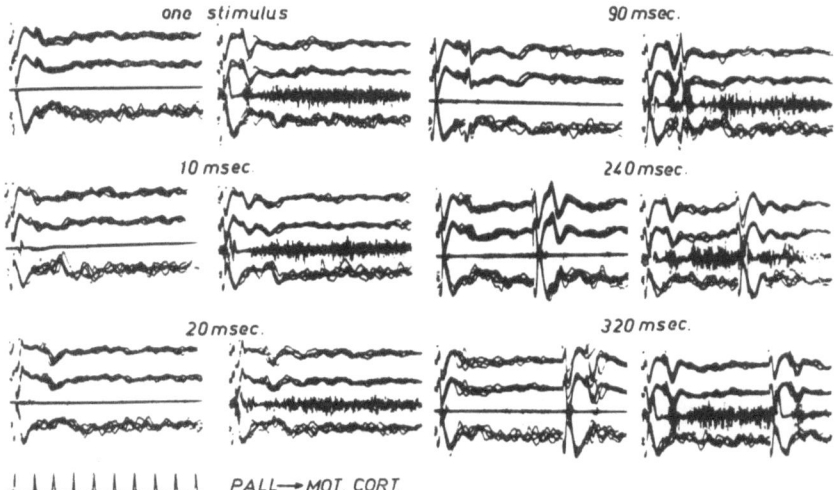

Fig. 2. Epilepsy. Stimulation of the right pallidum with single and double stimuli (15 V, 0.05 msec). Registration from three different point of the motor cortex on the same side and from the biceps muscle on the opposite side in rest and during voluntary contraction. With one stimulus one can see a pronounced functional dependency, it means, that during voluntary contraction the evoked potentials are enhanced especially a wave parallel with the peripheral motor rebound activity. At double stimulation with 20 msec distance between stimuli the evoked potentials in rest are very similar to the answers of one stimulus during voluntary contraction. At double stimulation with 240, 320 msec distances between stimuli the second evoked potential are more pronounced in rest but its functional dependency reversed to the first. The second answers with 320 msec distance between stimuli are not only more pronounced in rest as the first but parallel with the rebound wave (80 msec from the second stimulus) there is a group of electrical activity in the EMG. Calibration of amplitude: 0.05 mV in the EEG and 0.5 mV in the myogram

num, the postero-lateral and postero-medial nuclei of the thalamus and the mesencephalic reticular system. In this study we have used the double stimulation technique (DISA Multistim, 0.05–0.1 ms, 1–50 V square wave impulses, 0–400 ms distance between the two stimuli). We registered parallely the evoked potentials in different deep structures, in the cortex (from three different points of the same structure or of its surroundings) on the side of the stimulation (in the

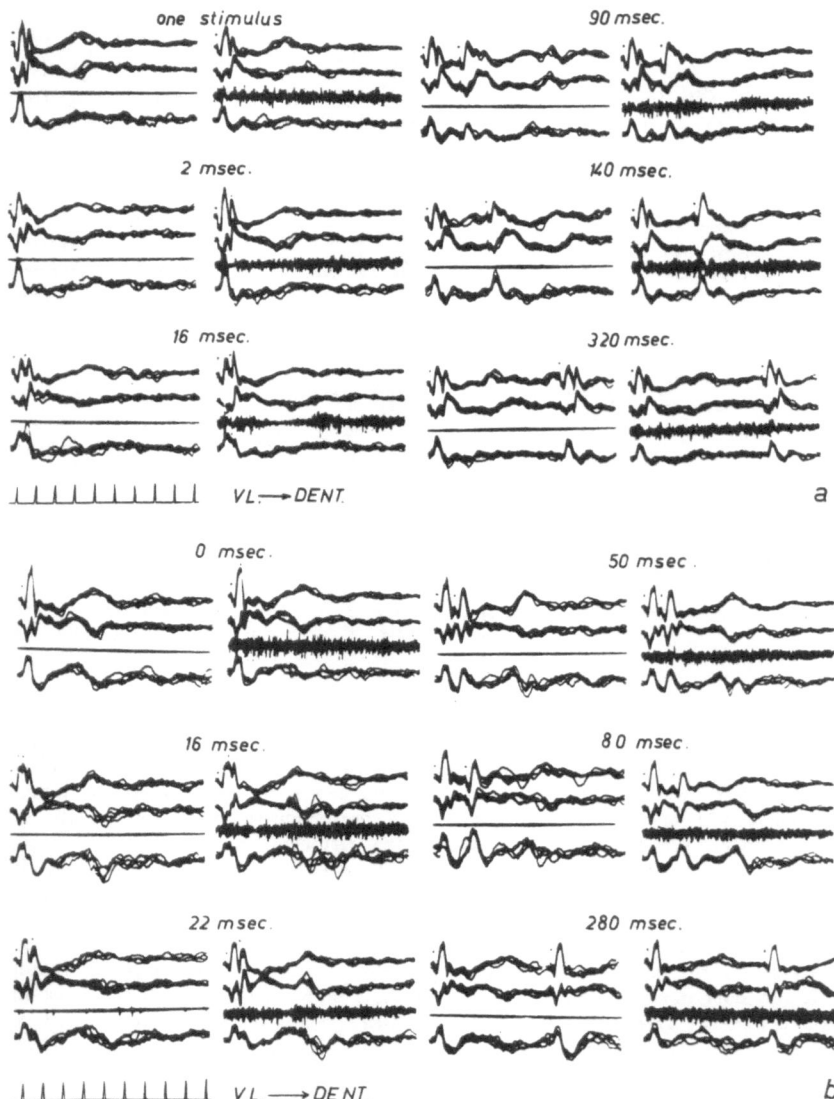

Fig. 3. a) The same patient as in Fig. 2. Stimulation of the posterior lower border of the right ventrolateral nucleus with single and double stimuli. Registration from three different point of the left brachium conjuctivum-dentate nucleus complex and from the left biceps muscle in rest and during voluntary contraction. The late component are pronounced in the evoked potentials, but especially longlasting changes are in the motor activity with a 16 msec distance between stimuli. b) Stimulation of the anterior upper border of the right ventrolateral nucleus with double stimuli. The late components are pronounced especially with 16.22 msec distances between stimuli. At the same time the functional dependency is high. Calibration of amplitude is the same

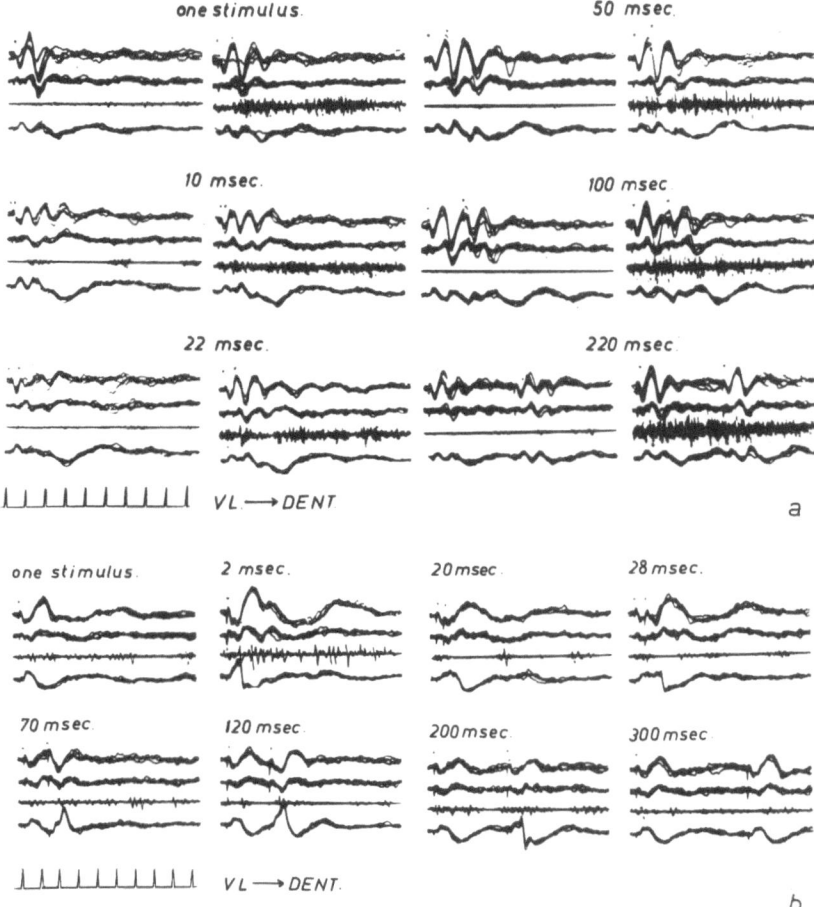

Fig. 4. a) Parkinsonism. Stimulation of the posterior lower border of the left ventrolateral nucleus with single and double stimuli (30 V, 0.05 msec). Registration from three different point of the right brachium conjuctivum-dentate nucleus complex and from the right biceps muscle. At the beginning the second stimulus destroys the evoked potentials of the first stimulus (10, 22 msec distances), than enhances it (50, 100 msec distances). At the 100 msec distance between stimuli the evoked potentials to the two stimuli look like as a whole in rest, but during voluntary contraction there are a clear separation between the two evoked potentials. b) Stimulation of the anterior upper border of the left ventrolateral nucleus with single and double stimuli (45 V, 0.05 msec). Registration as in a) in rest or with a little spontan tremor. Very clear the enhancing effect of the second stimulus (at 2, 20, 28 msec distances between stimuli). Very interesting the behaviour of the evoked potential on the fourth channel. This potential at 2 msec distance of stimuli appears in an enhanced form than disappears to the second stimulus. After a development appears again to the second stimulus in an enhanced form at 200 msec distance of stimuli, very probable with the 5 cps own rhythmicity of the motor system (5 cps tremor). Calibration of amplitude: 0.1 mV in the EEG and 0.2 mV in the myogram

dentate nucleus on the opposite side) and the motor answer on the opposite side (MEDICOR four channel registration equipment) in rest, and during voluntary contraction. On the record there are five to ten superimposed traces. It is natural that the first stimulus—within a time span—will influence the answer to the second stimulus but because of the longlasting evoked potentials and motor answers (especially during voluntary contraction) the second stimulus will influence the answer to the first, not as in the case of H-reflex recovery investigation.

We never found that the second evoked potential disappears. From this point of view it is not realistic to speak about recovery investigation, but it is wiser to speak only about the modification of the evoked potentials.

The answer of the double stimuli were analysed in rest and during voluntary contraction. The motor answer at the periphery during voluntary contraction was quite easily demonstrable but in rest we always choose the stimulus parameters so that a single stimulus never elicited motor answer. Anyway, the analysis of the answers of double stimulation is complicated, reflecting the complicated process itself.

Usually the evoked potential to one stimulus showed where we can expect the most pronounced changes to the second stimulus. On the Fig. 1 the second stimulus in 28 ms distance destroys the late component (rebound wave) of the first evoked potential correlating with the motor rebound activity. The second evoked potential and the motor answer become more pronounced and longer if the second stimulus is in the time of the rebound wave of the first evoked potential [90–100 ms distances between stimuli (Fig. 1)] correlating at the same time with the 10 cps rhythmic properties of the evoked rhythmicity on this patient (Tóth, Zaránd, and Lázár 1974).

Often one can not see the very late (over 100 ms) component of the evoked potential to one stimulus (Fig. 2) and only with double stimulation it is possible to detect the late changes, as in Fig. 2 with a 240, 320 ms distance between stimuli. At the same time the functional dependency of the second answer is reversed to the first. If we compare the former with another experimental situation within the motor system on the same patient (Fig. 3), one can see the very late component in the evoked potential and motor answer to a single stimulus. One can produce the same in an enhanced form by double stimulation with short distance between stimuli (Fig. 3 a and b; 16, 22 ms).

The double stimulation can enhance or depress the effect of a single stimulus with short distances between stimuli (0–100 ms)

(Fig. 4) with a longer distance between stimuli usually the consequences of the first stimulus will affect the answer to the second stimulus.

References

Tóth, Sz., Zaránd, P. (1972, 1973), Corticalis és subcorticalis ingerléseket követő reflexszerü izomválaszok emberen. Testneveléstudomány 1972/4—1973/1, 29—39.

— (1972), Effect of electrical stimulation of subcortical sites on speach and consciousness. Neurophysiology studied on man, pp. 40—46. Amsterdam: Excerpta Medica.

— Zaránd, P. Lázár, L. (1974), The role of the cortex and subcortical ganglia in the evoked rhythmic motor activity. Acta Neurochir. (Wien) 21, 25—33.

— — — Vajda, J. (1975), Effect of voluntary innervation on the evoked potential of the motor system. Confin. Neurol. (Basel) 37, 49—55.

— Vajda, J., Zaránd, P. (1976), The motor mechanism of some types of epilepsy. Acta Neurochir. (Wien), Suppl. 23, 51—57. Wien-New York: Springer.

Author's address: Sz. Tóth, M.D., National Institute of Neurosurgery, Budapest, Hungary.

Acta Neurochirurgica, Suppl. 24, 159—161 (1977)

Departments of Surgery and Neurostructure and Function, University of Texas
Medical School at Houston, Houston, Texas

Modification of Thalamic Evoked Activity
by Dorsal Column Stimulation

P. L. Gildenberg and K. S. K. Murthy

Recordings were made in two patients who had basal thalamotomies for intractable pain in whom, coincidentally, dorsal column
stimulators had previously been implanted in an unsuccessful attempt
to control their pain.

The lesion was produced in the intralaminar area according to
the method of Spiegel *et al.* (E. A. Spiegel, H. T. Wycis, E. G.
Szekely, P. L. Gildenberg, and C. Zanes: Combined dorsomedial,
intralaminar, and basal thalamotomy for relief of so-called intractable pain. J. Internat. Coll. Surg. *42*, 160–168, 1964).

One patient had post- amputation pain involving the right lower
extremity. The nature of the pain was both of a phantom type and
of burning dysesthesias over the stump. Much of the dysesthesia
followed an unsuccessful cordotomy for the treatment of phantom
limb pain. A dorsal column stimulator had previously been placed in
the upper thoracic area. Although the patient had the sensation of
stimulation into the area of pain and into the phantom limb, minimal
pain relief resulted.

The other patient suffered from post-laminectomy arachnoiditis.
He had had bilateral cordotomies, with post-cordotomy dysesthesia.
A dorsal column stimulator had been placed at the upper thoracic
level which gave relief of his pain only in the lowermost part of
his body. Consequently, a second dorsal column stimulator had been
placed in the lower cervical area. Coincidentally, one dorsal column
stimulator had been placed above the level at which the post-
cordotomy dysesthesia began and the other was placed below that
level.

Transcutaneous stimulation of the median and sciatic or sural
nerves was carried out in the operating room. Peripheral stimulation
was carried out bilaterally so that both ipsilateral and contralateral

evoked potentials could be recorded. Frequency varied from once per second to 0.2 per second and was delivered with a Grass S-4 Stimulator through an isolation unit. The peripheral stimulation was calibrated prior to surgery with a threshold to nonpainful and pain sensation. The stimulation in the levels affected by the cordotomy did not produce a painful sensation even at maximal setting of the stimulator.

Recording was done by means of a Spiegel-Wycis side-arm electrode. The signal was amplified and processed through a Nicolet 1072 computer. The raw data was simultaneously stored on magnetic tape for further processing later.

The dorsal column stimulator units were controlled with a special unit which allowed the stimulator to trigger the computer. Also, a wider variety of stimulus parameters was available than with the usual clinical unit. Stimuli to the dorsal column were applied first at a frequency of one to six per second for evoked potentials, and then the frequency with which the patient previously had experienced maximal pain relief was employed in an attempt to modify peripheral nerve evoked potentials.

Because of constraints imposed by minimizing the duration of the surgical procedure, to avoid unnecessary discomfort to the patient already under stress, and to avoid any electrode puncture of the brain which was not a necessary part of the surgical procedure, the manipulation for the sake of recording was minimized, sometimes at the expense of the quality of the recordings.

Single stimuli of the dorsal column stimulating electrode resulted in evoked potentials recorded in the intralaminar area. The initial wave of this response ocurred with an extremely short latency so that the calculated conduction velocity was about 200 meters per second. This was a consistent finding in both patients and on repeated stimulation. The authors have no indication of what pathways were involved with this very rapid conduction time. In the patient in whom two dorsal column stimulating electrodes had been implanted, an identical conduction velocity was calculated for both the upper and lower electrodes.

With an increase in the stimulus strength a very late negative wave appeared in the evoked potential with a latency of approximately 400 milliseconds.

Stimulation of the ipsilateral median nerve while recording with the tip of the side-arm electrode directed laterally toward the ventroposterolateral nucleus resulted in the appearance of a late component to the evoked potential as the stimulus strength passed the pain threshold. The addition of dorsal column stimulation during the peripheral nerve stimulation tended to return the later part of the wave form toward the control.

Stimulation of the contralateral median nerve while recording in the intralaminar nucleus resulted in the appearance of a large negative deflection with a latency of approximately 400 milliseconds as the stimulus exceeded the threshold for pain. This large negative depression was no longer seen when dorsal column stimulation was added.

Authors' address: P. L. Gildenberg, M.D., and K.S.K. Murthy, Departments of Surgery and Neurostructure and Function, University of Texas Medical School at Houston, Houston, TX 77025, U.S.A.

Acta Neurochirurgica, Suppl. 24, 163—173 (1977)
© by Springer-Verlag 1977

Stereotactic and Functional Neurosurgical Section of the Neurosurgical Clinic
(Prof. J. Bonnal), University of Liège, Belgium

Auditory Evoked Potentials Recorded
From Chronic Implanted Gyrus of Heschl in Man

A. Waltregny, F. Trillet, and A. Geurts

With 7 Figures

Summary

By means of implanted multileads electrodes, responses to clicks and prolonged sound stimulations were recorded from the Heschl gyrus of 2 human brains.
These responses were strictly localized to this structure. Cortical averaged auditory evoked potentials (c.AEP) to clicks are consistent with scalp averaged auditory evoked potentials (s.AEP). So, N_a, P_a, N_b, P_1, N_1, waves have similar
latencies and none of them in the s.AEP may be correlated with myogenic potentials (in opposition with the suggestions of Bickford et al. 1964 and Celesia et al.
1968). Increasing the duration of sound stimulation resulted in changes of the
response. For a duration longer than 20 ms, an "on-response" and an "off-
response" were noted. No satisfying physiological explanation of these events
is retained despite data obtained with monaural homo and heterolateral stimulations and with variation of tone of sound stimulation.

Key words: Auditory evoked potentials, depth chronic electrodes.

Introduction

It is now recognized that the human scalp recorded auditory
evoked potential (s.AEP) contains a sequence of 15 separate waves,
which is assumed to correspond with the activation of different
structures of the auditory pathway from brainstem to cortex (Picton
et al. 1974). These anatomical correlations were determined by
account of calculated latencies without any experimental confirmation.

There are few authors who have recorded evoked potentials to
click stimulation from the human cortex. The Rochester's school with
Sem-Jacobsen and Chatrian, was the first to present with depth
electrodes, records of responses of the human brain. In 5 patients,
the accidental placement of the multileads electrodes in the auditory

pathways permitted the direct electroencephalographic record of complex responses evoked by single clicks or repetitive clicks at low rate. For higher rates (more than 15 c/s) a sequence of three events was recognized an "on-response", a "driving response" and an "off response". These auditory responses decrease during pentothal

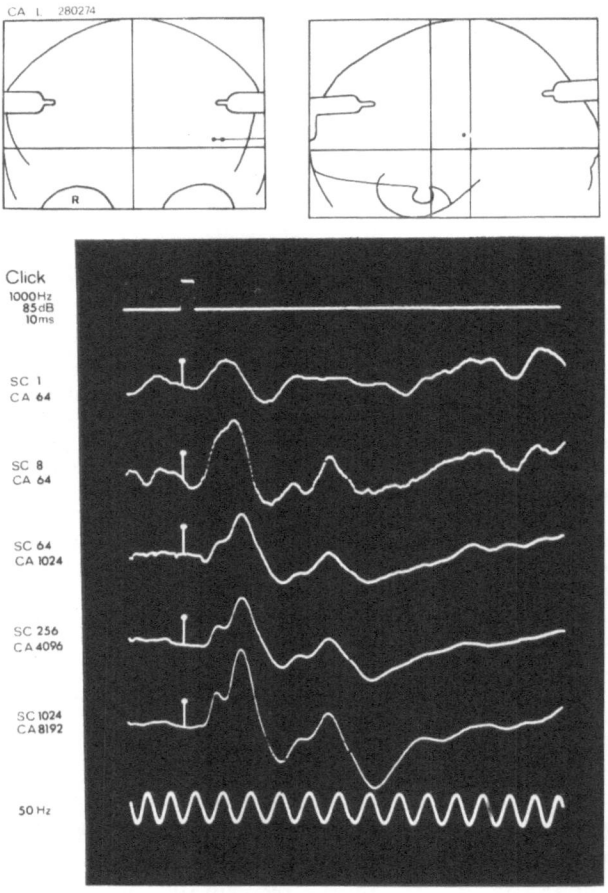

Fig. 1. The cortical averaged AEP to clicks. Progressive construction of the AEP from 1 (upper trace) to 1024 (lower trace) auditive short stimulations

anesthesia and the latency is longer in comatose patient. The driving response is recognized of lower voltage (about 85 per cent) when the homolateral ear is stimulated (Sem-Jacobsen *et al.* 1956, Chatrian *et al.* 1960).

The McGill's school using the cortex exposed ECoG technique of Penfield was able to determine the extent of superficial cortex activated by binaural acoustic stimuli.

6 fully conscious epileptic patients, the averaged cortical auditory evoked potentials (c.AEP) were recorded from the two upper

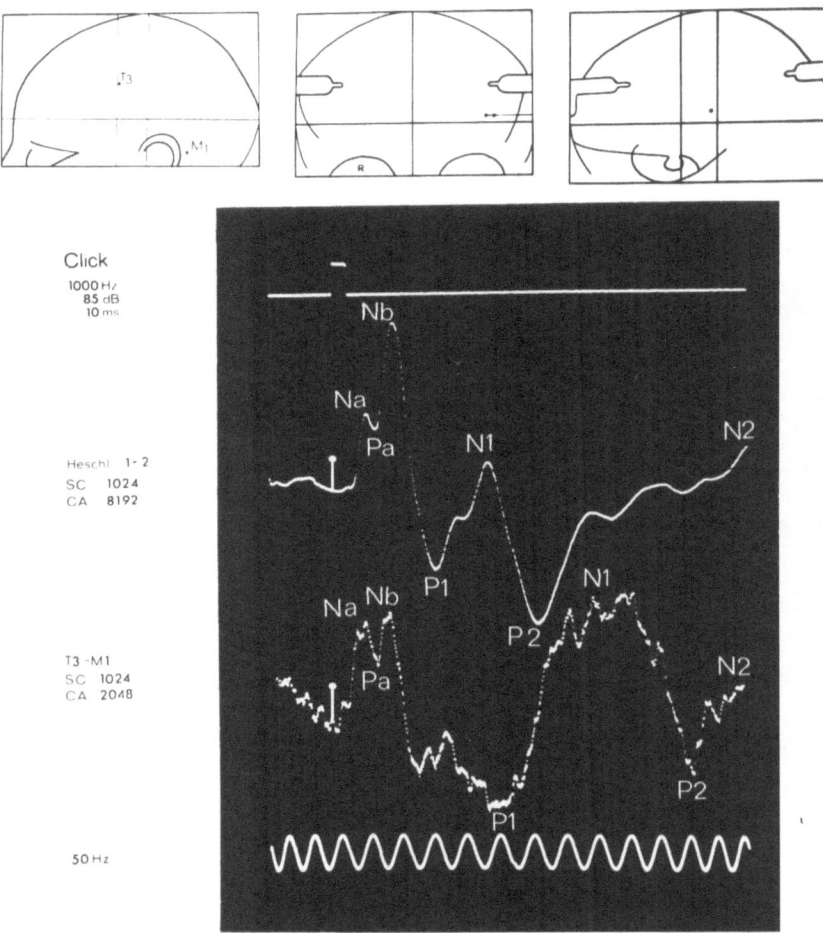

Fig. 2. The cortical and scalp averaged AEP to clicks. Simultaneous scalp and cortical AEP. The short latencies deflections are quite similar, but the tardive waves are delayed on the scalp

and lower posterior banks of the sylvian fissure. The authors considered that the summated responses were originated in the Heschl gyri and transmitted by volume conduction to the adjacent gyri,

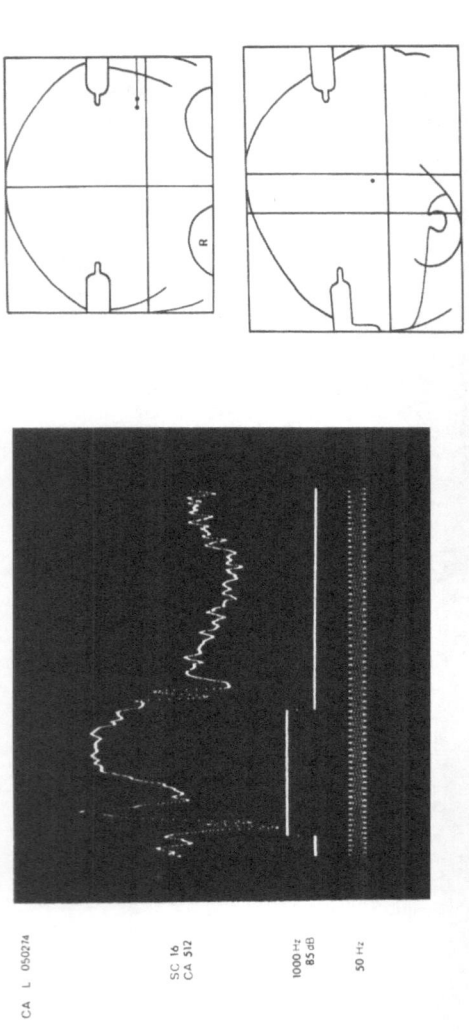

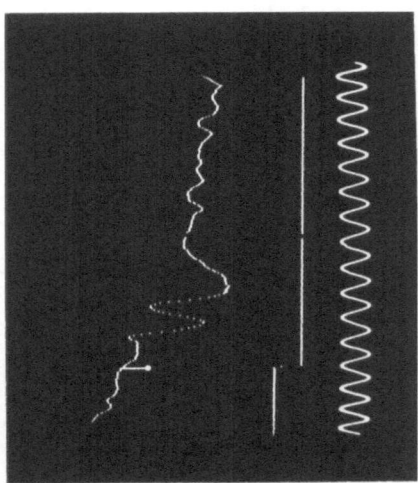

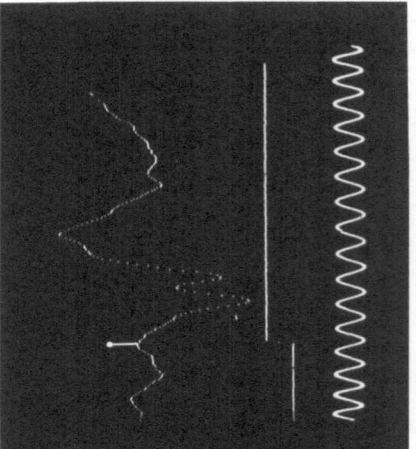

Fig. 3. The cortical averaged AEP to prolonged sound. With an auditive stimulation as long as 400 ms, an "on-response" and an "off-response" are clearly recognizable (upper trace). With the X-axis extension, the latencies of the initial deflec-

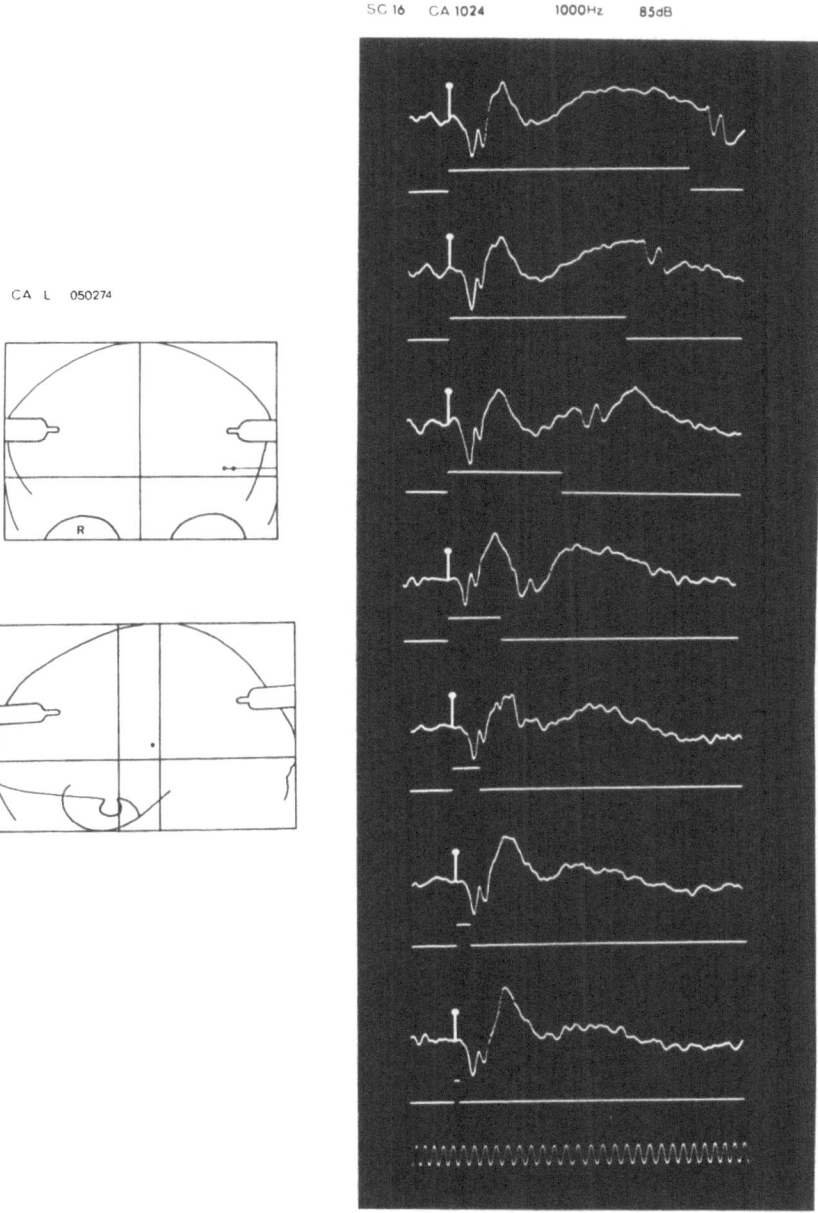

Fig. 4. The cortical averaged AEP to sounds with different durations. The progressive reduction of the duration of the auditive stimulation from 880 ms to 10 ms shows the progressive imbrication of the "off" in the "on-response"

but direct recording from the superior surface of the temporal lobe
was not carried out (Celesia *et al.* 1968). Using our own chronically
implanted multileads electrodes technique, we were able to study the
c.AEP to various monaural and binaural auditive stimulations.

Methods

Patients. This study is based on observations made in 2 patients. One
had a left temporal epilepsy and several multileads electrodes were implanted
in the temporal lobe including the Heschl gyrus with regards to auditory epileptic
hallucinations. The second patient had a right infantile hemiplegia and the
chronic SEEG examination was carried out before cortical excision. These
technical and methodological procedures were carried out under the most rigourous
aseptic techniques and our primary consideration was to the patients welfare
according to the ethical principles of the declaration of Helsinki (1964).

Location of responsive electrodes. According to the arteriographic visualization
of the transverse temporal gyrus, the multileads gold electrodes were precisely
implanted with the Talairach's stereotaxic system (Talairach *et al.* 1967). The
electrodes are fixed on the skin and are soldered to one or two 44 MMS 127-
Metrelec®-miniature connectors fixed on the scalp with stainless steel wires. Each
lead is 0.2 mm in diameter and 4 mm long; the distance between several contacts
on the electrode is 4 mm. The final diameter of the electrode is from 1 to 1.8 mm
according to the number of leads.

Stimulation and recording. Auditory stimulations are obtained by feeding the
rectangular pulses of a Wavetek (Model 112) clock-timed with a Grass S 88
stimulator, to a stereo earphones set. Monaural or binaural stimulations are presented randomly every 3–5 s according to the duration of these stimulations.
The patient is sitting in a soundattenuated room. The bipolar inputs from the
electrodes are led into a Elema-Schönander electroencephalograph with output to
a 8-channel 6,200 PI tape recorder and to a 4-channel 1,000-BIOMAC analyzer
with a 502 A-TEKTRONIX oscilloscope. The prepulse from the stimulator is
used to trigger the analyzer.

Scalp averaged auditory evoked potentials are recorded simultaneously with
gold skin sutured electrodes. The sound parameters are 10 ms to 1 s in duration,
100 Hz to 7,000 Hz, and 60 to 90 dB.

Results

Responses to click. The bipolar response to a binaural single
click (1,000 Hz, 10 ms) evoked from a waking patient, is recognized
as a gross-biphasic potential. The latencies of the initial and the
second deflections are respectively about 35 ms and 60 ms (Fig. 1).
The averaging of repetitive clicks shows the construction of a more
complex potential variation (Fig. 1). For a large number of sweep
counts, it is possible to recognize a succession of waves of which
calculated latencies indicate a good correlation with the successive
deflections of the s.AEP. The latencies of the different waves are
respectively 25, 45, and 105 ms for one polarity, and 30, 70, and
130 ms for the other polarity. This waves are assumed to cor-

respond respectively to N_a, N_b, N_1 and to P_a, P_1, P_2 of the Davis' nomenclature and Picton's works (Fig. 2).

Responses to sound. When the duration of the auditive stimulation is increasing, new phenomena appear (Fig. 3). While a large evoked potential is detected immediately after the beginning of the

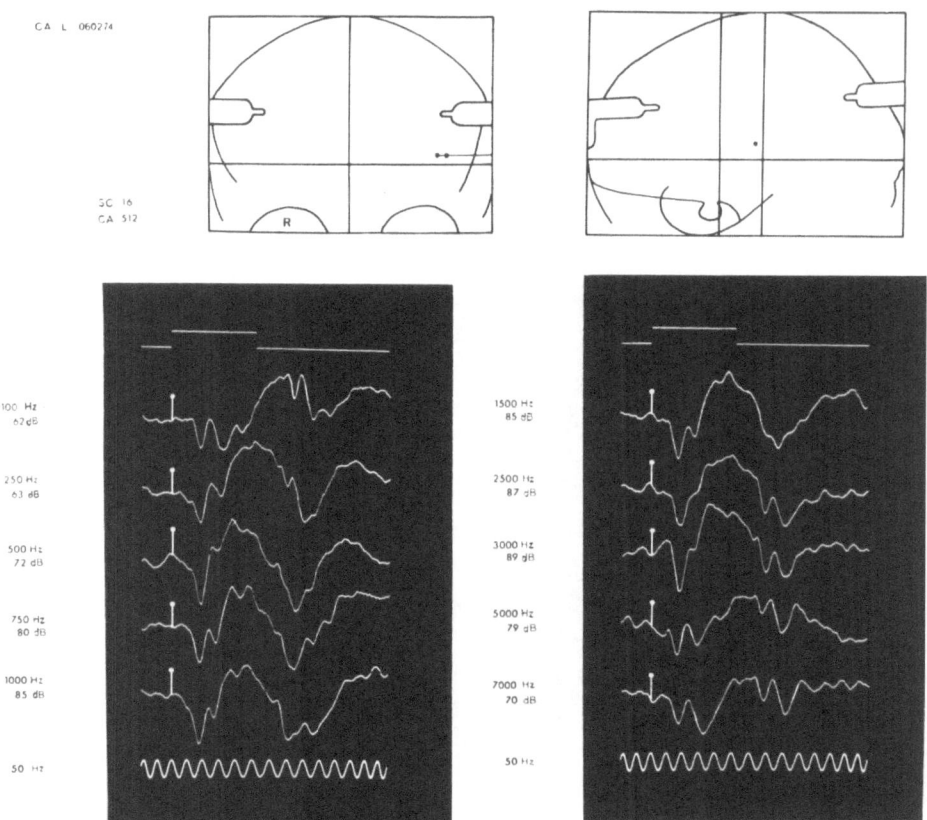

Fig. 5. Variation of the cortical averaged AEP with the frequency of the auditive stimulation. The frequency of the sound is growing up from 100 Hz to 7,000 Hz. Note the modifications of the slow waves

auditive stimulation, one other but lower is present after the end of the sound presentation. In fact, these "on" and "off" potentials are perfectly superposable. The N_a, N_b, P_a, P_1, N_1 deflections have the same latencies with regards to the beginning and the end of the sound stimulation. This "off" potential appears to interfer with the tardive slow deflection of the "on potential". This is particularly evident when the duration of the sound stimulation is progressively reduced (Fig. 4). For short presentations, "on" and "off" responses are imbricated. This interference is present for duration of sound longer than 20 ms (Fig. 4).

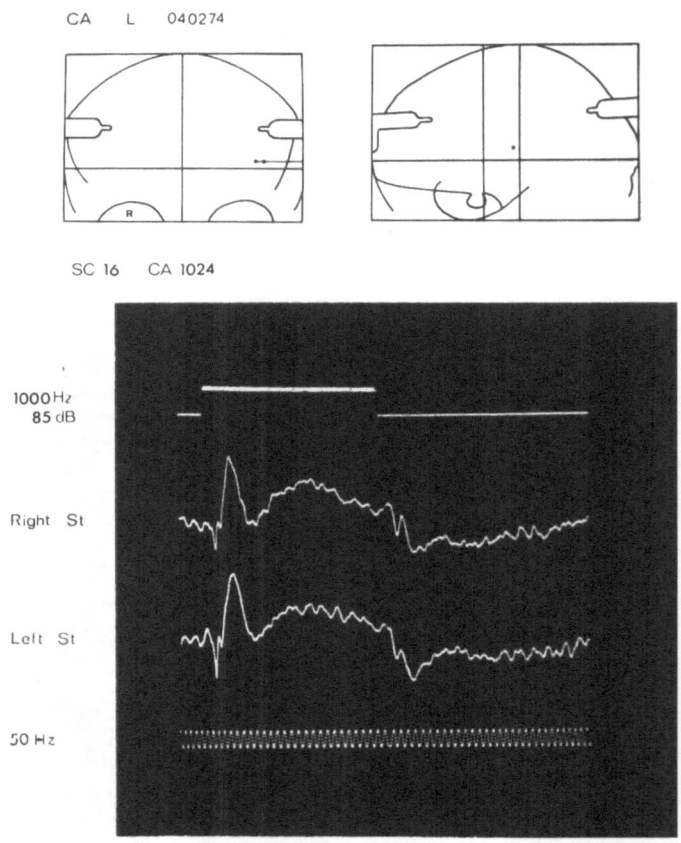

Fig. 6. Left AEP to right and left monaural stimulations. Note the similarity of the AEP despite the different conditions of acoustical stimulations

The pattern of the evoked response is modified when the frequency of the sound stimulation increases. The major change touchs the large slow wave N_2 (Fig. 5). This wave is more tardive in the low frequencies and its relative amplitude decreases for sounds with frequency higher than 5,000 Hz. The practical consequence of this phenomenon is a better visualization of the "off" response to stimulations at high frequency with respect to the decrease of the interaction between the "on" and "off" potentials (Fig. 5).

*Responses to homo- and heterolateral monaural sound stimbla-
tions.* In the lesion-free awake subject, the complex sequence of
potentials does not change with the left or right monaural acoustic
stimulation (Fig. 6).

Comparative responses of left and right Heschl gyri. In the
infantile hemiplegic patient, the comparative study of electrical
responses of the left and the right gyri demonstrates a significant

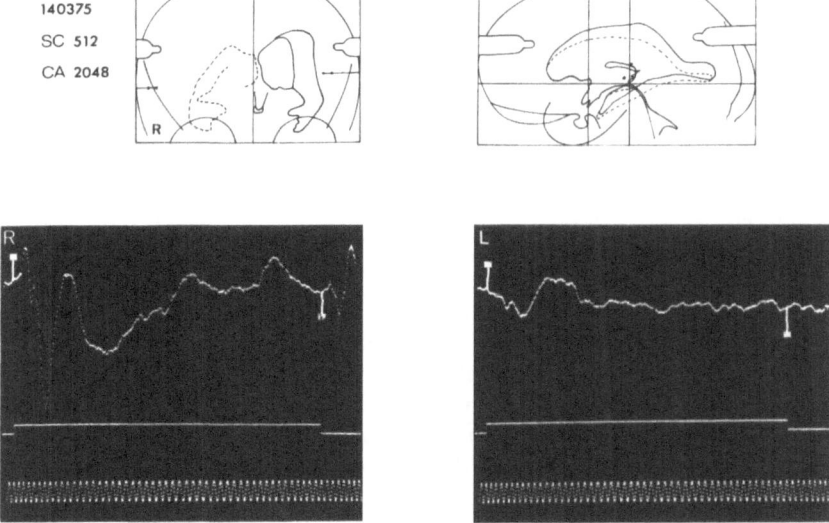

Fig. 7. Comparative AEP on the normal and damaged cortex. Note a good AEP
on the normal Heschl gyrus (*R*) with "on" and "off-responses". On the damaged
Heschl gyrus (*L*) the "on-response" is significatively attenuated and no "off-
response" is detected

lower voltage in the damaged cortex. Furthermore, the off-potential
is not recognized in this same cortex although he is present in the
normal gyrus (Fig. 7).

Comment

The cortical responses to single and repetitive clicks, and to
prolonged sound stimulations were not frequently studied in man
principally because of the limitations intrinsic to human experimenta-
tion. Undoubtly, the opportunity to have chronic multileads electrodes implanted in Heschl gyri of epileptic patients, is quite un-
common. This explains the rareness of results about this physiological
question.

Thus in our 2 patients, we have recorded single sweep responses from the Heschl gyrus. The *biphasic* response to a single click has latencies which agree with those described by Chatrian *et al.* (1960) and Celesia *et al.* (1968). It is an interesting fact to notice that our results are obtained with short distance bipolar records; this strengthens the located origin of these potentials over the risk to introducing volume conducted events with the averaged technique.

Such summating technique permits a good extraction of the different components of the c.AEP. Evaluating respective latencies, it is possible to recognize their valuable correspondance with the N_a, P_a, N_b, P_1, P_2, and N_2 waves of Picton's works. Furthermore, our results demonstrate the reality of the cerebral origin of all these s.AEP's components. Increasing the duration of the sound stimulation up to 20 ms produces a more complex response which may be separated between an "on" and an "off-response". These potentials are not different from the "on" and "off-responses" recognized by Chatrian *et al.* (1960) at the beginning and at the cessation of a clicks' train at relatively high rate (up to 15 c/s). Our data indicate:

1. "on-response" and "off-response" are quite similar (Fig. 3);
2. they are identical to the single click evoked potential (Fig. 2);
3. they are resembling to the evoked responses to paired clicks (Chatrian *et al.* 1960). It is thus interesting to notice that a similar but opposite sense sudden change of noise (installation or suppression) may produce an identical complex variation of potential (on-, off-response). It is not easy to think that these evoked potentials are really evoked by the volley of neuronal afferences since no potential may be recorded in the auditory nerve at the time of cessation of an auditive stimulus. Of course a good alternative for a physiological explanation may be that the major part of these potentials would be a neuronal cortical reaction to the acoustical messages assuming that the brutal interruption of significant stimulus may be interpreted as the audition of resting noise. Unfortunately, they are no experimental physiological data about such hypothesis. On the other hand, it may be possible to consider that these "on" and "off" responses are unspecific potentials to the auditive stimulation in a psychophysiological point of view. Chatrian *et al.* (1960) pointed out that either type of "on" and "off response" may be absent or rather unconspicuous while the other is well developped. In the same way, they are significatively decreased during anesthesia and coma. Recently Cooper presented some records in which some similar c.AEP are detected in the frontal lobe of neurotic patients on psychosurgical treatment (Pfurtscheller and Cooper 1975). However, we must note that we were not able to record such similar potentials in

other sites of the temporal lobe including middle and inferior temporal gyri, hippocampus and amygdala. Two other points are unrelated with a such unspecific interpretation; they are 1. the variation of slow waves with the frequency of sound stimulation (Fig. 5); 2. the stability of such responses at intervals below 500 ms. But on the other hand in the normal cortex, these potentials are not different after monaural homo- and heterolateral stimulations. Thus some considerations but not all are consistent with the unspecific hypothesis but this remains to be clearly determined.

References

Bickford, R. G., Jacobson, J. L., Cody, D. T. (1964), Nature of averaged evoked potentials to sound and other stimuli in man. Ann. N.Y. Acad. Sci. *112*, 204—218.

Celesia, G. G., Broughton, R. J., Rasmussen, T., Branch, C. (1968), Auditory evoked responses from the exposed human cortex. Electroenceph. clin. Neurophysiol. *24*, 458—466.

Chatrian, G. E., Petersen, M. C., Lazarte, J. A. (1960), Responses to clicks from the human brain. Some depth electrographic observations. Electroenceph. clin. Neurophysiol. *12*, 479—489.

Davis, H., Yoshie, N. (1963), Human evoked cortical responses to auditory stimuli. Physiologist *6*, 164.

— Zerlin, S. (1966), Acoustic relations of the human vertex potential. J. acoust. Soc. Amer. *39*, 109—116.

Declaration of Helsinki (1964), Recommandations guiding doctors in clinical research. Wld. med. J. *2*, 281.

Pfurtscheller, G., Cooper, R. (1975), Selective averaging of the intracerebral click evoked responses in man: an improved method of measuring latencies and amplitudes. Electroenceph. clin. Neurophysiol. *38*, 187—190.

Picton, T. W., Hillyard, S. A., Krausz, H. I., Galambos, R. (1974), Human auditory evoked potentials. Evaluation of components. Electroenceph. clin. Neurophysiol. *36*, 179—190.

— — (1974), Human auditory evoked potentials. Effects of attention. Electroenceph. clin. Neurophysiol. *36*, 191—199.

Sem-Jacobsen, C. W., Petersen, M. C., Dodge, H. W., Lazarte, J. A., Holman, C. B. (1956), Electroencephalographic rhythms from the depths of the parietal, occipital and temporal lobes in man. Electroencephal. clin. Neurophysiol. *8*, 263—278.

Talairach, J., Szikla, G., Tournoux, P., Prossalentis, A., Bordas-Ferrer, M., Covello, L., Iacob, M., Mempel, E., Buser, P., Bancaud, J. (1967), Atlas d'anatomie stéréotaxique du télencéphale. Paris: Masson.

Waltregny, A., Trillet, F., Petrov, V. (1975), SEEG et gyrus cingulaire normal. Acta Neurol. Belg. *75*, 113.

Authors' address: Waltregny, A., M.D., Dr. Sc., Neurosurgical Clinic, University of Liège, Boulevard de la Constitution 66, B-4000 Liège, Belgium.

Acta Neurochirurgica, Suppl. 24, 175—178 (1977)
© by Springer-Verlag 1977

Department of Neurological Surgery, Kantonsspital, University of Zürich,
Switzerland

The Effect of Graded Thermocoagulation on Trigeminal Evoked Potentials in the Cat

G. Broggi and J. Siegfried

Since Sweet's proposal in 1969 [16] of using radiofrequency (RF) current heating to coagulate trigeminal retroganglionar fibers for treatment of trigeminal neuralgia, quite a few reports [3, 10, 11, 12, 13, 14, 15] have been published confirming the success of such a surgical technique.

All the authors made the clinical observation that analgesia can be achieved without any or with minimal tactile sensitivity defects.

The RF current effect is due to the heat generated through the tissues [2]: the clinical results suggest that, as for local anesthetics [7], a different sensitivity to graded heating does exist between large and small diameters nerve fibers.

But to date no physiological or histological ground has been found for this selectivity of action of the RF current on nerve fibers, except for one *in vitro* study on the isolated saphenous nerve of the cat. Lecther and Goldring [9] have indeed been able to show a non-linear relationship between fibers diameters and sensitivity to RF current in the peripheral nerve.

The aim of this study was to determine the existence of a similar relationship among the trigeminal nerve fibers.

Method

Twelve adult cats anesthetized with Pentrane and paralyzed with succinyl-choline after Ketamine anesthesia induction, underwent open surgery. Tracheostomy and hemicraniectomy were performed, the tentorium was removed and, after hemicerebellectomy, the gasserian ganglion and the trigeminal nerve were exposed with the use of an operative microscope.

A concentric bipolar stimulating electrode was inserted into the pulp cavity of an ipsilateral tooth. Supramaximal stimulus strenght was employed (3 to 9 V; 0.5 msec duration; 1/sec to 100/sec frequency). Evoked potentials or single unit activities have been recorded from the retroganglionar trigeminal fibers through a tungsten microelectrode completely isolated except for the final 10–15 microns of the tip, measuring 1–2 micron in diameter, against a reference electrode placed in the frontal bone. The evoked responses were displayed in the AC coupled channel of an oscilloscope after passing through a short and long time constant amplifier.

When a clear response was evoked a probe (n. 18 gauge needle, with insulated shaft and exposed tip) was inserted in the gasserian ganglion distally to the recording electrode, and graded RF current was applied. The termistor housed into the probe allowed, through a Wheatestone bridge, determination of the temperature reached in the trigeminal fibers. The presetted temperature was maintained for 60 seconds.

At the end of the experiments the animals were killed with an overdose of barbiturate (Nembutal) and the trigeminal nerve was dissected free for electrode positions checking and for histological and electron microscopy examination.

Results

A compound action potential has always been evoked in response to 0.5 ms square wave electrical pulses delivered to tooth pulp, in the ipsilateral retroganglionar trigeminal fibers.

The analysis of this compound action potential permitted the identification of different components. Because of the relationship between nerve fibers diameter and conduction velocity of nerve impulses [7], the various components are due to different size axons excitation. A alpha, A delta, and C fiber potentials have been identified, with a conduction velocity respectively of 70 m/s, 21 to 11.20 m/s, and 5.60 to 1.40 m/s. Such values are in agreement with those proposed by Darian Smith et al. [5], Andersen and Pearl [1], and Grubel [8].

When RF current was applied to the gasserian ganglion while a compound action potential was evoked in the retroganglionar fibers, the response seemed to be modified as soon as 45 °C were reached. Further graded RF current heating produced clearcut variations in the compound action potential profile: at 45 to 50 °C, A delta fibers potentials was decreased more than the C fibers one, while the A alpha one showed no variation. When 60 to 65 °C has been maintained for 60 seconds, the A delta and C fibers components were abolished, with little or without any alteration of the earlier components of the compound action potentials. Over 65 °C also A alpha fibers components consistently decreased in amplitude: nevertheless in some experiments also at 45 °C temperature these fibers became affected. Single units discharges of C fibers were affected at 45 to 50 °C.

When abolished, the responses did not reappear even after 120 minutes recovery intervals.

Discussion

Our results demonstrate that the compound action potential, because of its latency, its configurations, its ability to follow up high frequency stimulation (65/s), should be due to orthodromically conducted nerve impulses in the trigeminal fibers, and that the late responses are not due to trigeminal dorsal root reflex [4, 6].

Furthermore we can now assume that RF current affects trigeminal nerve fibers with a non-linear relationship between axons diameter and temperature reached: indeed A delta fibers showed in many cases a critical temperature to RF current effect lower than any other trigeminal nerve fibers. C fibers only some times were affected at the same temperature than A delta fibers.

But it must be remarked that the differential critical range of temperature is very narrow (5 to 8 °C) for C fibers and A delta fibers, while A alpha fibers are consistently affected by the RF heating only at greater temperature (over 65 °C).

Since neurosurgeons very frequently experience in their clinical practice that 65 °C is a critical temperature to achieve analgesia avoiding any major tactile defect, it does not seem hazardous to put forword the hypothesis that human trigeminal nerve fibers behave during RF current heating the same as cat trigeminal nerve, and that a few minutes of such a procedure give long lasting A delta and C fibers impairment and is the reason for long lasting analgesia in patients. Our results do not explain why A delta fibers seem to be affected before C fibers, in accord with Letcher and Goldring [9] observations on the isolated saphenous nerve.

The possibility of blocking in a definite manner nerve impulse conduction in fibers carrying sensitive impulses of different modality, substanciates clinical results in trigeminal neuralgia treatment.

References

1. Anderson, K. V., Pearl, G. S. (1974), Conduction velocities in afferent fibers from feline tooth pulp. Exp. Neurol. *43*, 281—283.
2. Aronow, S. (1960), The use of radio-frequency power in making lesions in the brain. J. Neurosurg. *17*, 431—438.
3. Broggi, G., Thermorhizotomy in trigeminal neuralgia: preliminary considerations upon 46 cases. Proc. Congr. German Neurosurg. Soc., Heidelberg, May 1975. In: "Advances in Neurosurgery". Berlin-Heidelberg-New York: Springer. In press.
4. Darian, Smith I. (1966), Neural mechanisms of facial sensation. Inter. Rev. Neurobiol. *9*, 301—395.
5. Darian, Smith I., Mutton, P., Proctor, R. (1965), Functional organization of tactile cutaneous afferents within the semilunar ganglion and trigeminal spinal tract of the cat. J. Neurophysiol. *28*, 682—694.

6. Frigyesi, T. L., Broggi, G., Siegfried, J. (1975), Evoked potentials in the trigeminal dorsal root: their selective vulnerability to graded thermocoagulation. Expt. Neurol. *49*, 11—21.
7. Gasser, H. S., Erlanger, J. (1929), The role of fiber size in the establishment of a nerve block by pressure or cocaine. Amer. J. Physiol. *88*, 581—591.
8. Grubel, G. (1970), The physiology of single neurons of the trigeminal nuclei. In: Trigeminal neuralgia (Hassler, R., Walker, E. A., eds.), pp. 73—83. Stuttgart: G. Thieme.
9. Lecther, F. S., Goldrings, S. (1968), The effect of radiofrequency current and heat on peripheral nerve action potential in the cat. J. Neurosurg. *29*, 42—47.
10. Nugent, R. G., Berry, B. (1974), Trigeminal neuralgia treated by differential percutaneous radiofrequency coagulation of the gasserian ganglion. J. Neurosurg. *40*, 517—523.
11. Onofrio, B. M. (1975), Radiofrequency percutaneous Gasserian ganglion lesions. J. Neurosurg. *42*, 132—139.
12. Siegfried, J. (1973), Un nouveau traitement neurochirurgical de la nèvralgie du trijumeau: analgesie sans anesthésie. Neuro-Chirurgie *19*, 585—587.
13. Sweet, W. H., Wepsic, J. G. (1974), Controlled thermocoagulation of trigeminal ganglion and rootlets for differential destruction of pain fibers. Part 1: trigeminal neuralgia. J. Neurosurg. *39*, 143—156.
14. Tew, J. M. J., Mayfield, F. M. (1973), Trigeminal neuralgia: a new surgical approach. Laryngoscope *83*, 1096—1101.
15. Turnebull, I. M. (1974), Percutaneous rhizotomy for trigeminal neuralgia. Surg. Neurol. *2*, 385—389.
16. White, J. C., Sweet, W. H. (1969), Pain and the neurosurgeon: a forty years experience, pp. 184—197. Springfield, Ill.: Ch. C Thomas.

Authors' addresses: G. Broggi, Division of Neurosurgery, Istituto Neurologico, Milano, Italy, and J. Siegfried, M.D., Department of Neurological Surgery, Kantonsspital, University of Zürich, Rämistraße 100, CH-8091 Zürich, Switzerland.

Acta Neurochirurgica, Suppl. 24, 179—185 (1977)
© by Springer-Verlag 1977

Institute of Neurosurgery, School of Medicine, University of Buenos Aires,
Buenos Aires, Argentina

Functional Exploration of the Spinomedullary Junction

J. R. Schvarcz

With 4 Figures

The application of percutaneous and stereotactic techniques to
the spinal cord has opened an exciting new field, which has provided
a unique opportunity to study—with therapeutic purposes—the functional organization of the spinomedullary region.

However, there are many challenging problems still unsolved.
Stereotactic spinal surgery presents particular problems of its own.
In contrast to the relative immobility of the intracranial structures,
the cord is freely mobile within the spinal canal. Nevertheless, its
displacement can be largely restricted by the axial elongation
produced by full ventroflexion of the head (Breig 1960). A certain
degree of rotation is unavoidable, and is related to the selected
track and target (Hitchcock 1972 b).

Within the small confines of the cord, the tiny size of the target,
its complex spacial evolution and the important surrounding structures, as well as their anatomical variation, must be accounted for.
We could improve and sophisticate the mechanical and radiological
accuracy of the technique, but still anatomical variation will need
to be individually evaluated, a fact which is sometimes overlooked.

In this respect, I would like to comment on a case I have recently
operated on: it was a spinothalamic tractotomy in which, from
3 different parallel tracks, only ipsilateral responses were obtained.
Finally, I decided to explore the other side of the cord. At target,
ipsilateral paresthesiae were easily elicited in the painful sacro-
lumbar distribution, and a lesion produced a dense ipsilateral analgesia. It was, most probably, an uncrossed spinothalamic tract, a fact
already well documented (French and Peyton 1948, Voris 1951,
White and Sweet 1969).

Hence, we must not forget that what gives spinal cord stereo-

12*

tactic techniques their particular benignity is precisely the fact
that they are performed in an alert, cooperative patient, thus
allowing—and demanding—an adequate electrophysiological corroboration of the target site. So far, this can be accomplished by
impedance measurement, electrical stimulation, depth recording and

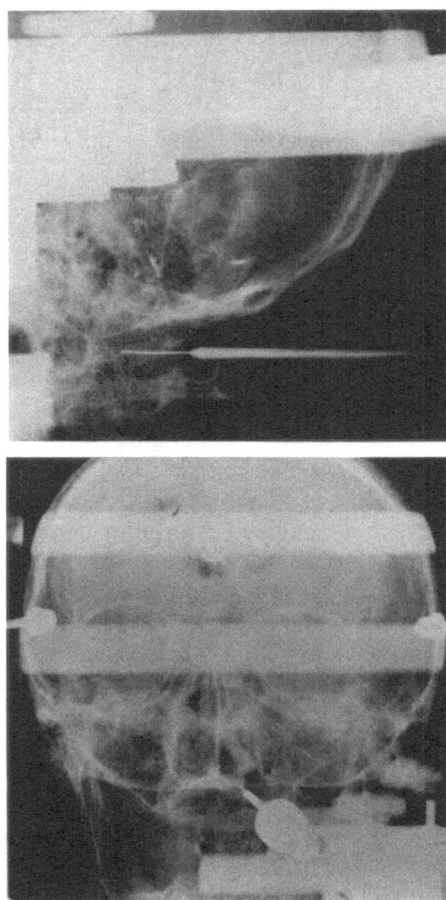

Figs. 1 and 2. Lateral and anteroposterior radiographs with the electrode in place
showing the posterior atlontooccipital approach

incremental enlargement of the lesion with concomitant clinical
testing. Avoidance of any of this essential steps will unduly increase
the hazards of the procedure and will further compromize its effectiveness.

Material and Methods

The technique and the indications, contraindications and limitations for each particular procedure have already been reported (Schvarcz 1974, 1975, 1976), and will not be further elaborated here. I shall only point out that the spinomedullary region was always stereotactically approached by a posterior track through the atlontooccipital space (Figs. 1 and 2), as proposed by Hitchcock (1972 b), with a tungsten electrode of 0.5 mm diameter, with a 2 mm bare end electrolytically sharpened, which allowed recording, stimulation and destruction.

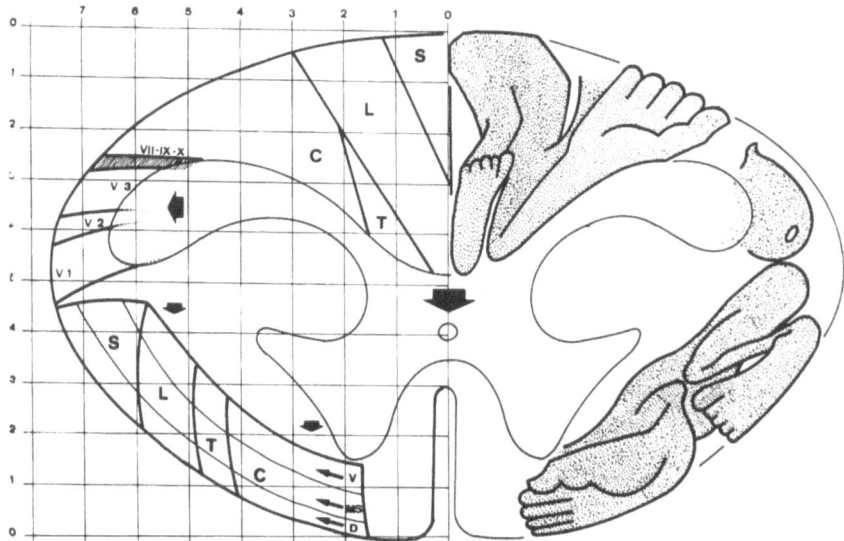

Fig. 3. Functional map of the high cervical cord. At the right, the classical dermatomal representation; at the left, the homuncular arrangement proposed in the text

The medial region was explored during extralemniscal myelotomy, the lateral region during trigeminal nucleotomy, and both during spinothalamic tractotomy.

Since a particular response can be due to stimulation of any one of a number of different sites, the whole track lenght was routinely explored.

1905 stimulation responses from 100 consecutive operations, representing 127 tracks, were plotted and referred to cord contact, and correlated with the data available from depth recording and incremental destruction. A tentative map was thus outlined (Fig. 3).

Results

The dorsal column has a definite homuncular arrangement, which allowed an accurate lesion siting for myelotomy. This implies the existance of a dorso-ventral topical organization, combined with the commonly recognized mediolateral lamination of the funiculus.

Provided that a midsagital track was used, sensory responses from both lower limbs were consistently elicited, with the representation of the distal parts located deeper, towards the central canal, and with the fibers from the dorsal segments of the limb lying on the central septum. This arrangement fits in with Hitchcock's findings (1972 a, b). This is not so, however, for the lateral region, mainly with respect to the position of the hand representation, which Hitchcock locates deeply, near the base of the posterior column and lateral to the foot area. Curiously enough, the whole disposition except for the hand representation is different from that reported by Hosobuchi *et al.* (1971).

Depth recordings only showed, so far, an increase of both the frequency and amplitude of the background activity, which was elicited by joint movement.

From the central canal region, a basic pattern of responses was consistently elicited (Schvarcz 1976), probably related to stimulation of the base of the dorsal funiculi. They consisted of paresthesiae which started at the soles of both feet and were propagated to the dorsal aspect of the legs with increased intensity of stimulation. This basic pattern could be obtained alone or with some additionally superimposed responses, such as trigeminal paresthesiae (usually involving its whole distribution), or less frequently, crossed limb involvement. They were regarded as due to stimulation of decussating fibers.

Other peculiar though inconstant responses were also elicited from this area: nausea, dizziness, respiratory changes (apnea with low frequency stimulation, and hyperpnea with higher frequencies) and sometimes, bilateral burning truncal sensations.

No modality difference was detected at different depths within the dorsal funiculus, at least by subjective sensations.

A single small destruction in this central cord region has produced striking effects, in ill accordance with established knowledge (Hitchcock 1970 a). Remarkably, both upper and lower body pain were easily dealt with by such a lesion, including central pain phenomena. I have stated that this is not a segmental, commissural procedure, but presumably it is related to the interruption of a multisynaptic non-specific asceding system (Schvarcz 1974, 1976). Pain relief was usually obtained without producing sensory losses. However, in the cases were it did occur, they had a rather bizarre distribution and furthermore, they could not be correlated with the presence or absence of pain.

At high C 1 level, responses from all the Vth. nerve divisions, including the circumoral fibers, were consistently elicited, as well as from the VIIth/IXth/Xth component. They followed the classical onion skin pattern, with the rostral dermatome located ventrolaterally, and the caudal one placed dorsomedially, just lateral to the VIIth/IXth/Xth fibers (Hitchcock 1970 b, Schvarcz 1975). It was possible to further define the dorsal border of the trigeminal area by the homolateral responses obtained from the cuneatus, and its ventral border by the contralateral responses elicited from the spinothalamic tract or, less commonly, by

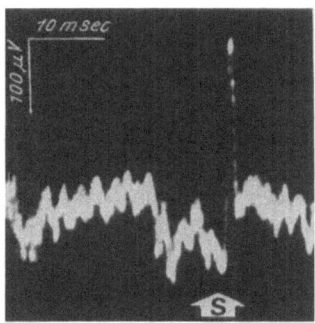

Fig. 4. Recording from the spinal trigeminal nucleus: evoked potential elicited by nociceptive stimulation

the motor responses produced from a posteriorly located corticospinal tract.

Sensations were also referred to the C 1-C 2 territory. Indeed, it was easy to obtain wide areas of analgesia, down to and including the C 2 dermatome, which demonstrated the extensive overlap of facial and cervical afferents at this level (Hitchcock and Schvarcz 1972).

At a very low C 1 level, however, central face responses were not constant or were obtained only with high voltages.

On depth recordings, nociceptive stimulation produced evoked potentials, which were elicited from very restricted ipsilateral fields (Fig. 4).

Both depth recordings and incremental coagulation suggested that the mucous surfaces are represented deeper than the skin, but at the same segmental level of the corresponding dermatome.

The functional exploration of the anterolateral funiculus has confirmed the classical somatotopic pattern of the spinothalamic tract. However, it has a definite homuncular arrangement, as first proposed by Hitchcock (1972 a, b), with the big hand and foot lying superficially. This was consistently confirmed by careful exploration of the whole track: *e.g.*, knee-elbow-hand is a common sequence (Schvarcz 1974).

In some cases, ipsilateral responses were also elicited. They were referred symmetrically but felt with less intensity than the concomitant contralateral sensations (Tasker *et al.* 1974). They were probably due to stimulation of uncrossed spinothalamic fibers, and perhaps they could explain the bothersome allochestesia which sometimes immediately followed lesion making.

Fractional incremental coagulation suggested that within the tract there is a clear lamination, with the dermatomal component superficially placed (Schvarcz 1974). This would explain why stereotactic lesions so often do not produce dense skin analgesia, but only of the deeper structures (Gildenberg 1972), in contrast with open techniques.

Motor responses (1–5 Hz, 0.5–1 volt) were generally obtained medially, from the decussation itself, or laterally, from the corticospinal tract. There is much variation in the size and position of the motor decussation (Taren *et al.* 1969). It occurs over 1 cm, between the obex and C 2, where the corticospinal tract assumes its final posterolateral position, with the upper extremity fibers medially, and the lower ones laterally and dorsally located.

The arm fibers cross more rostrally than the leg fibers do, and sometimes they were quite posteriorly and medially placed, a fact to be considered during myelotomy. There is also considerable variation in the direct corticospinal tract, though sometimes definite neck and shoulder responses were obtained. Segmental responses were obtained from a wide area, both medially and laterally, probably by stimulation of root fibers or anterior horn cells.

Only by strict adherence to the principles of physiological confirmation of the electrode placement will the effectiveness of these procedures be increased and their hazards be minimized. Furthermore, this will additionally result in a better and rewarding understanding of this complex region.

References

Breig, A. (1960), Biomechanics of the central nervous system. Stockholm: Almqvist and Wiksell.

French, L. A., Peyton, W. T. (1948), Ipsilateral sensory loss following cordotomy. J. Neurosurg. *5*, 403—404.

Gildenberg, P. L. (1972), Physiologic observations concerned with percutaneous cordotomy. In: Neurophysiology studied in man (Somjen, G., ed.), pp. 231 to 236. Amsterdam: Excerpta Medica.

Hitchcock, E. R. (1970 a), Stereotactic cervical myelotomy. J. Neurol. Neurosurg. Psychiat. *33*, 224—230.

— (1970 b), Stereotactic trigeminal tractotomy. Ann. Clin. Res. *2*, 131—135.

Hitchcock, E. R. (1972 a), Electrophysiological exploration of the cervico-medullary region. In: Neurophysiology studied in man (Somjen, G., ed.), pp. 237—245. Amsterdam: Excerpta Medica.

— (1972 b), Stereotaxis of the spinal cord. Confin. Neurol. (Basel) 34, 299—310.

— Schvarcz, J. R. (1972), Stereotactic trigeminal tractotomy for postherpetic facial pain. J. Neurosurg. 37, 412—417.

Hosobuchi, Y., Adams, J. E., Weinstein, P. R. (1971), Preliminary percutaneous dorsal column stimulation prior to permanent implantation. In: Proceedings, American Association of Neurological Surgeons.

Schvarcz, J. R. (1974), Spinal cord stereotactic surgery. In: Recent progress in neurological surgery (Sano, K., Ishii, S., eds.), pp. 234—241. Amsterdam: Excerpta Medica.

— (1975), Stereotactic trigeminal tractotomy. Confin. Neurol. (Basel) 37, 73—77.

— (1976), Stereotactic extralemniscal myelotomy. J. Neurol. Neurosurg. Psychiat. 39, 53—57.

Taren, J. A., Davis, R., Crosby, E. C. (1969), Target physiologic corroboration in stereotactic cervical cordotomy. J. Neurosurg. 30, 569—584.

Tasker, R. R., Organ, L. W., Smith, K. C. (1974), Physiological guidelines for the localization of lesions by percutaneous cordotomy. Acta Neurochir. (Wien) Suppl. 21, 111—117.

Voris, H. C. (1951), Ipsilateral sensory loss following cordotomy: report of a case. Arch. Neurol. Psychiat. 65, 95—96.

White, J. C., Sweet, W. E. (1969), Pain and the neurosurgeon. A forty years experience. Springfield, Ill.: Ch. C Thomas.

Author's address: Dr. J. R. Schvarcz, Las Heras 2012, Buenos Aires 1127, Argentina.

Acta Neurochirurgica, Suppl. 24, 187—190 (1977)
© by Springer-Verlag 1977

Institute of Neurology, Madras Medical College, Madras, India

Role of the Amygdala and Hypothalamus in the Control of Gastric Secretion in Human Beings

B. Ramamurthi, M. Mascreen, and K. Valmikinathan

Stereotaxic surgery on the human being, is an important field of activity at the Institute of Neurology, and surgery for behaviour disorders includes making lesions in the amygdala and in the hypothalamus. During surgery, the concerned deep nuclei of the brain are stimulated to ascertain the situation of the electrodes. This opportunity has been utilized to note the effect of stimulation of the amygdala and the hypothalamus on the production of acid in the stomach.

From animal experiments it is known that gastric secretions are influenced by higher neural mechanisms situated in the amygdala and the hypothalamus. Results of such stimulation are not available in the human subjects, as these operations are performed only in a few centres in the world.

Sub-cortical areas have long been known to react to stimulation by increasing gastric acidity. Porter *et al.* (1953) made an extensive study of the mechanisms by which hypothalamic stimulation increased acidity and found that this could occur not only via the vagal nerves but also via the pituitary and adrenal glands. A remarkable fact is the considerable latency of the change in the acidity (1 to 2 hours). According to the authors the results were reliable and could be repeated. Shealy and Peele (1957) found that stimulation of the amygdala in the unanaesthetized animals causes a definite increase in gastric acid content which compared favourably with the increase in acidity caused after histamine alone. These authors assumed that the effect of stimulating the amygdaloid nuclei could be mediated via histamine or via parasympathetic fibres in the vagus nerve. The pathways involved between the amygdaloid nuclei and the vagus nuclei remain unknown; it is possible that the connections between the amygdaloid nuclei and the hypothalamus may lead to activation of the hypothalamic area. Varieties of changes in gastric secretions were obtained by Anand, Dua, and Chinna (1957) on stimulation of temporal lobe structures with indwelling electrodes in unanaesthetized cats. These authors considered the possibility that this effect is transmitted through the hypothalamus.

It is thus clear that autonomic influences control the production of gastric acidity and such influences are under the control of higher centres, acting through the limbic systems and the hypothalamus. The medial part of the posterior hypothalamus is concerned with sympathetic discharges while a few millimeters lateral, stimulation is known to produce parasympathetic effects. With this knowledge in mind, gastric secretion was measured before, during and after making lesions in the amygdala and in the hypothalamus. In the amygdala the stimulation was mainly in the basolateral portion, the site at which the subsequent lesion was made. In the hypothalamus 2 sites were chosen for stimulation 1. the medial part of the posteromedian hypothalamus where a lesion was made subsequently and 2. a site 4 mm lateral to the target mentioned in (a).

A total number of 140 subjects drawn from the inpatients of the Institute of Neurology, taken up for stereotaxic surgery formed the group of the present study. Subjects posted for amygdalotomy and hypothalamotomy formed the study group while these posted for thalamotomy, cingulumotomy, dentatectomy, and leucotomy were studied as controls.

The Ryle's tube was introduced before the patient was anaesthetized for surgery. The correct position of the tube in the stomach was checked by routine radiological screening. Continuous aspiration of gastric contents was ensured by using a vacuum aspirator. Occasionally hand suction was also applied.

The pooled samples of gastric juice aspirated up to stimulation of the subcortical area formed the "pre-stimulation sample". The material collected between the time of stimulation and the time of making the lesion formed the "post stimulation sample". This period ranged between 30–45 minutes. Similarly samples of gastric juice collected 2 hours after the lesion were termed as "post-lesion sample". Post-lesion samples were also obtained 24 hours after the lesion.

The samples of gastric juice were analysed for free hydrochloric acid and total acid concentration. Aliquots of the centrifuged gastric contents were titrated against 0.01 N Sodium Hydroxide using Topfer's reagent and Phenolphthalein as indicators. The results of free acid and total acid were expressed as milliequivalents per litre.

Observation

The mean figures of total acid during prestimulation post-stimulation and post-lesion periods of the control and study groups are presented in Table 1.

Table 1. *Mean Values of Total Acid During Pre Stimulation,*
Post Stimulation and Post Lesion Periods

	No. of cases studied	Total acid before stimulation M.Eq/1	Total acid after stimulation M.Eq/1	Total acid 2 hours after lesion M.Eq/1
Amygdalotomy	49	128.9 ± 23	164.6 ± 17.4	96.8 ± 13.6
Hypothalamotomy	33	100.7 ± 26.4	121.2 ± 18.4	90.9 ± 22.6
Thalamotomy	33	57.7 ± 26.6	56.7 ± 23	49.43 ± 12.6
Cingulumotomy	15	50.5 ± 13.1	80.4 ± 15.4	75.4 ± 15.6
Dentatectomy	10	40.9 ± 7.8	52 ± 9.6	45.3 ± 9.7
Total	140			

This shows that:

1. The initial gastric acid level was found to be high in the majority of patients who underwent amygdalotomy or hypothalamotomy. The cases chosen for other types of stereotaxic surgery, and used as controls, exhibited a lower initial gastric acid level.

2. Stimulation of the amygdala and hypothalamus leads to a significant increase in the total acid secretion.

3. Two hours after making the lesion there is a fall in the acid secretion to a level lower than the initial values.

Table 2. *A Study of Gastric Secretion During Stereotactic Amygdalotomy*

49 cases		
Increase in acid on stimulation 65% *	No change on stimulation 3%	Fall in acid on stimulation 32% **
Increase in acid ——— after lesion 3%	(2 cases showed fall in acid after lesion)	Fall in acid ——— after lesion 58%
Fall in acid after lesion 97%		Increase in acid after lesion 38%

* 65% of cases showed increase in acid after stimulation. The mean figures of acid of these cases are:

Before stimulation	*After stimulation*	*After lesion*
156	232.9	126.8

** 32% of cases showed a fall in acid after stimulation. The mean figures of acid (M.Eq/1) of these cases are:

86.8	54.0	51.8

An analysis of the amygdalotomy cases shows that there are 2 distinct groups of cases 65% with high initial acid levels and 35% with lower levels. The response to stimulation in these cases varied. The cases with initial high acid level showed marked increase of acid on stimulation whereas the ones with low initial acid showed a fall in acid levels on stimulation. All cases however showed a fall in acid level after the lesion.

A study is now being conducted to correlate the clinical picture and the response to surgery of these two different groups of patients.

In the hypothalamotomy cases, a lower initial acid level was seen only in 2 patients.

A comparison of the stimulation effects of medial and lateral hypothalamus showed that the acid level almost always increased after stimulation of the lateral area. This is in conformity with our known knowledge that this area is concerned with parasympathetic activity. However it is to be noted that stimulation of the medial hypothalamus also caused elevation of gastric acid levels in a number of patients. This may mean that the medial hypothalamus is not purely sympathomimetic.

Lesions in the medial hypothalamus resulted in a less marked reduction in gastric acid secretion compared to the amygdala. No lesions were made in the lateral part of the hypothalamus in any case as there was no therapeutic indication.

One may conclude that the amygdala and the hypothalamus have a role in determining human gastric acid secretion levels. The mechanisms of such action cannot be determined by human experiments as such clinical situations do not exist. As a corollary it is to be investigated whether initial gastric acid values and the responses obtained on stimulation and after the lesion may be taken as a guide to prognosis in such cases and also for selecting suitable cases for sedative neurosurgery.

References

1. Anand, D. K., Dua, S., Chhina, G. S. (1957), Changes in the behaviour produced by lesions in the frontal, and temporal lobes. The Ind. J. Med. Research *45*, 3, 353—357.
2. Porter, R. W., Movius H. J., French, J. D. (1953), Hypothalamic influences on hydrochloric acid secretion of the stomach. Surgery *33*, 875—880.
3. Shealy, C. N., Peele, T. L. (1957), Studies on amygdaloid nucleus of cat. J. Neurophysiol. *20*, 125—139.

Authors' addresses: B. Ramamurthi, Professor of Neurosurgery, Neurosurgeon and Head of the Department, Institute of Neurology, Madras Medical College, Madras-3, India; M. Mascreen, Junior Research Fellow, University Grants Commission, Institute of Neurology, Madras Medical College, Madras-3, India; and K. Valmikinathan, Professor of Neurochemistry, Institute of Neurology, Madras Medical College, Madras-3, India.

Acta Neurochirurgica, Suppl. 24, 191—198 (1977)
© by Springer-Verlag 1977

Department of Neurobiology, Max-Planck-Institut für Hirnforschung,
Frankfurt/M., Federal Republic of Germany

The Effects of Drugs on the Field Potential
in the Caudate Nucleus Following Nigra Stimulation

A. Wagner, M. Dupelj, and K. C. Lee

With 3 Figures

The reciprocal connections of the caudate (Cd) and nigra (Ni) nuclei have been extensively studied using anatomical [2, 17, 26, 27, 28, 35, 36, 37], histochemical [1, 13, 30, 8] and electrophysiological [3, 6, 9, 12, 14, 15, 22, 23, 24, 38] methods but in some respects the situation is even less satisfactory than a few years ago. The present communication is aimed at examining the characteristics of field potentials in the Cd evoked from stimulation of the Ni before and after systemic application of drugs. The cats were anaesthetized with sodium pentobarbital (30–40 mg/kg), immobilized by flaxedil and artifically ventilated. The overlying cortical structures were removed by suction to expose the dorsal surface of the Cd. The nigro-caudate pathway was electrically stimulated using bipolar electrodes placed in the Ni proper. Similar electrodes in the cerebral peduncle (CP) allowed antidromic activation of the Cd. Field potentials were recorded in the medial two thirds of the ipsilateral Cd with glass microelectrodes filled with either 2 M sodium chloride or 3 M potassium chloride (DC resistance: 3–5 MΩ). A Nicollete 1074 was used for averaging the signals. The recording and stimulating electrode tracts were identified histologically.

Fig. 1 A illustrates the nature of the field potential recorded at different depths in the caudate following nigra stimulation. This consisted of a negative wave with superimposed spike discharges followed by a slow positive potential. The negative wave had a mean latency of 12 msec and a duration of 8 msec. This pathway conducts impulses slowly (0.9–1.1 msec) and excites a characteristic population of cells distributed throughout all regions of the caudate. This orthodromically activated wave is always the earliest recordable

event. Therefore it is most likely that the negative wave results from
action potential and synaptic currents of the activated Cd neurons.
From this evidence it seems likely that all inputs into the Cd are
excitatory. The slow positive wave had an average latency of
20 msec and a duration of 50–70 msec. This positivity increases with
the depth of penetration of the electrode. The fibres from the nigra
tend to form contacts with the dendritic and spinous fields of caudate
neurons, suggesting that many neighbouring cells are contacted by

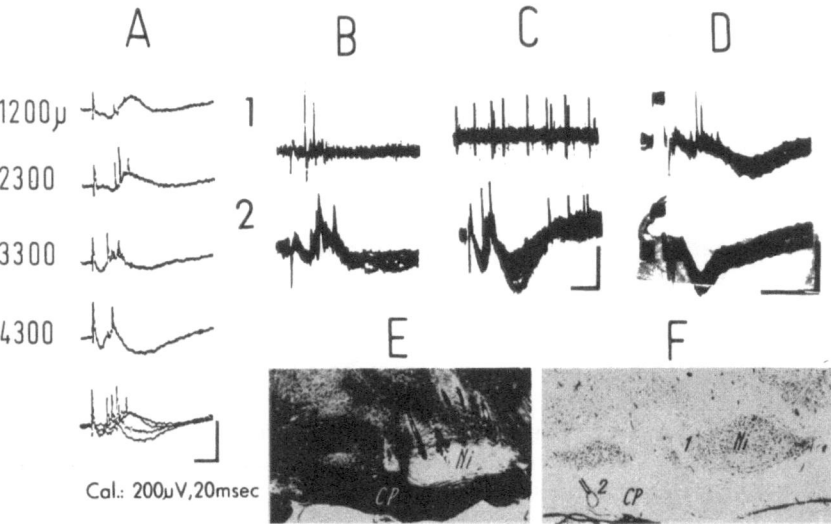

Fig. 1. Field potentials recorded in the Cd following Ni stimulation. A) Recorded
from different depths along the microelectrode tract. Last picture in A represent
all superimposed sweeps. E) Histological identification of the position of stimulating
electrodes for A. In B 1 extracellular records of excitation of silent Cd cells by
Ni stimulation. B 2 corresponding field potential. C 1 spontaneous active cell in Cd
and C 2 corresponding field potential. D 1 orthodromically activated field. D 2 antidromic evoked positivity. F) The position of stimulating electrodes for D. Stimulus
intensity 10 V. Cal: 200 µV, 20 msec

the same fibres. One could assume that inhibitory cells surrounding
the monosynaptically activated cells are also activated by nigra
stimulation, thus generating the inhibitory slow potential. This
could represent one type of inhibition. In E the position of
stimulating electrodes is shown. The characteristic excitatory ortho-
dromic response of silent cells in the Cd to nigral stimulation is illustrated in Fig. 1 B 1 and in B 2 is the corresponding field potential.
Microiontophoretic injection of dopamine (DA) has no effect on
these cells. Conversely, for the spontaneous active caudate cell shown

in C 1, it can be observed that the spontaneous firing was silenced during the slow positive phase of the field potential (C 2). The spontaneous activity of Cd cells can be blocked by the iontophoretical application of DA. The cessation of firing could have been also produced by other events (disfacilitation or excessive depolarisation).

Shown in D 1 are the well known field potentials resulting from Ni stimulation. The second spike superimposed on the negativity always disappeared after *i.v.* injection of 10 mg/kg sodium pento-

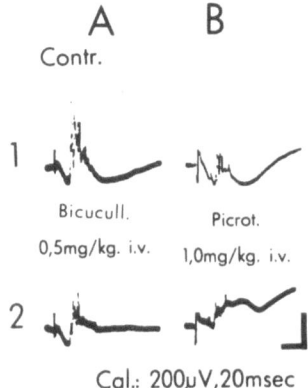

Cal.: 200µV, 20msec

Fig. 2. The effect of systemically administrated drugs on the field potential in Cd following Ni stimulation. A_1 and B_1 control records of field potential in two different experiment. A_2 after systemic application of 0.5 mg/kg bicuculline *i.v.* and B_2 after administration of 1.0 mg/kg picrotoxin. Single stimulus, intensity 10 V, was the same with control and after administrated drugs. Cal: 200 µV, 20 msec

barbital and/or 25 mg/kg mephenesin, suggesting that they may be polysynaptic in nature (not shown in picture). In D-2 the anti-dromic stimulation in the peduncle only produces a positive wave. The conduction velocity of ortho- and antidromic impulses are the same. The fact that the wave following antidromic stimulation is a positive one indicates that the recording electrode is not located near GABA-ergic cells. In F the position of stimulating electrodes is shown. Since the possibility of recurrent inhibition by way of axon collaterals exists, it is tempting to speculate that the slow positive wave recorded in the Cd may be GABA-ergic in nature.

Bicuculline suppresses a number of synaptic inhibitions suspected of being mediated by GABA. When administered iontophoretically, bicuculline selectively reduces the inhibitory effect of GABA. But bicuculline seems also to be moderately potent competitive inhibitor of brain ACh-E [34]; bicuculline might influence some function of the cholinergic system. After application of 0.5–1.0 mg/kg bicuculline *i.v.* (Fig. 2 A 2), the negativity was unchanged, but the positive wave was selectively and reversibly blocked. In B 2, the injection of 1.0 mg/kg picrotoxin even reverses the polarity of the positive wave. The substance amino oxyacetic acid (AOAA), an inhibitor of GABA-transaminase, increases the GABA concentration in the CNS. One hour after *i.v.* administration of AOAA at 10.0 mg/kg (Fig. 3 A 2), the positive wave was clearly increased. Presumably, the increase in the positive field is related to the known increase in GABA concentration. There is no change in the negative wave. The caudate and putamen are one of the brain structures richest in acetylcholine (ACh) and their related enzymes, acetylcholinesterase (ACh-E) and choline transferase (ChAc), and also have the highest catecholamine concentration. The interruption of nigro-striatal connexions leads to an inbalance between ACh and DA. This can be produced with 6 hydroxy dopamine (6-OH-DA) which induces selective degeneration of catecholamine nerve terminals in the brain and a marked increment of ACh level in the caudate. This increase is produced through the inhibition of ACh-E in the striatum [20]. A similar antagonistic relation between DA and ACh content has been found by hemilesion experiments [16]. The concentration of ACh in the Cd is dependent on the DA input; however, GABA-ergic neurons in the striatum are not affected by 6-OH-DA.

After *i.v.* application of reserpine, we had no selective change in the field potential. Administration of 100 mg/kg L-Dopa causes only a minimal increase in the polysynaptic input. It becomes interesting, then to know whether the GABA-ergic component of the field potential is affected when the concentration of ACh is enhanced. After intra-carotid injection of 0.1 mg/kg of ACh, the field potential shows no change in negativity, but the positive wave is blocked (Fig. 3 B 2). The mechanism, which this occurs is not clear.

In Fig. 3 C we show the results of the action of haloperidol on excitatory synaptic input and positive wave. Kim and Hassler [21] have demonstrated, that haloperidol significantly decreases the GABA level but not the GAD and GABA-T activity in the striatum and nigra. With application at 2.0 mg/kg *i.v.* of haloperidol (Fig. 3 C 2), the negative wave as well as positive wave are blocked. The absence of a negative wave might result from an action on the dopaminergic pathway or receptor. It could be a non-specific type of neural depression [4]. The blockage of the positive wave results from an increase of ACh, or an absence of DA, or the direct blockade of GABA.

Normal relations of the basal ganglia involve a coordinated functioning of different groups of neurons whose transmitters are GABA, DA, ACh, and their related enzymes. The Ni is normally influenced and controlled by the striatum. Strio-nigral fibres to the pars reticulata and pars compacta seem to be GABA-ergic because the GABA concentration in the nigra, which is the highest in the brain, drops by nearly 2/3 after interruption of the strio-nigral fibres [16, 19, 33] and the pleomorphic type of axodendritic synapses in the nigra degenerates [10]. Neurophysiological studies have demonstrated a distinct inhibitory

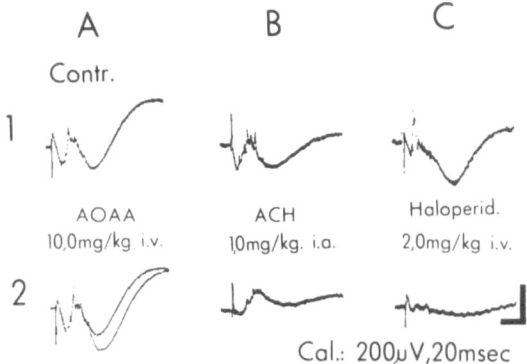

Fig. 3. The effect of systemically applied drugs on the field potential in Cd evoked by single stimulus in Ni. A_1, B_1, C_1 control field potentials in three different experiments. A_2 60 min after 10 mg/kg *i.v.* bicuculline. B_2 15 min after 1.0 mg/kg *i.v.* ACh and C_2 90 min after 2 mg/kg *i.v.* haloperidol. Stimulus 10 V 0.1 msec. The voltage calibration represent 200 µV, time 20 msec

effect [38] of the Cd on the Ni which is blocked by picrotoxin [31]. Also, the iotophoretic application of GABA clearly depresses the firing rate of Ni cells [7]. More recently Okada and Hassler (1973) experiments have demonstrated that GABA is released from isolated slices of rat Ni by electrical stimulation. DA is released in the striatum from cells originating in Ni and may either excite or inhibit striatal neurons. Our experimental data show that the stimulation of the Ni produces excitatory mono- as well as polysynaptic responses in Cd.

It is possible that these excitations are product of the non-dopaminergic pathway from the Ni to the Cd. Monosynaptic excitation in Cd by Ni stimulation can also be triggered in the absence of a dopaminergic innervation [5]. A second type of Cd neurons, "spontaneously active", are blocked either following Ni stimulation or after iontophoretically applied DA. If the positive field are rearly produced through the GABA-ergic collaterals, ACh plays a very important role as the antagonistic interrelation of GABA output. For the Cd to function normally it is necessary to maintain a balance between ACh and GABA output, as well as a normal level of DA input. It seems that most neurological and mental disorders may be produced by disturbances in GABA output.

References

1. Anden, N. E., Carlsson, A., Dahlström, A., Fuxe, K., Hillarp, N. A., Larsson, K. (1964), Demonstration and mapping out of nigrostriatal dopamine neurons. Life Sci. (Oxford) *3*, 523—530.
2. Bak, I. J., Choi, W. B., Hassler, R., Usunoff, K. G., Wagner, A. (1975), Fine structural synaptic organization of the corpus striatum and Substantia Nigra in rat and cat. Advances in Neurology, Vol. 9, pp. 25—41. New York: Raven Press.
3. Feltz, P., Albe-Fessard, D. (1972), A study of an ascending nigro-caudate pathway. Electroenceph. clin. Neurophysiol. *33*, 179—193.
4. Feltz, P. (1971), Sensitivity to haloperidol of caudate neurones excited by nigral stimulation. Europ. J. Pharmakol. *14*, 360—364.
5. Feltz, P., Champlain, J. de (1972), Persistence of caudate unitary responses to nigral stimulation after destruction and functional impairment of the striatal dopaminergic terminals. Brain Res. *43*, 595—600.
6. Feltz, P., McKenzie, J. S. (1969), Properties of caudate unitary responses to repetitive stimulation. Brain Res. *13*, 612—616.
7. Feltz, P. (1970 b), Relation nigro-striatale: essai de différentiation des excitation et inhibition par micro-iontopharèse de dopamine. J. Physiol. (Paris) *62*, 151.
8. Fibiger, H. C., Mc. Geer, E. G., Atmadja, S. (1973), Axoplasmic transport of dopamine in nigro-striatal neurons. J. Neurochem. *21*, 373—385.
9. Frigyesi, T. L., Purpura, D. P. (1967), Electrophysiological analysis of reciprocal caudato-nigral relations. Brain Res. *6*, 440—456.
10. Hajdu, F., Hassler, R., Bak, I. J. (1973), Electron microscopic study of the Substantia Nigra and the strio-nigral projection in the rat. Z. Zellforsch. *146*, 207—221.
11. Hassler, R., Wagner, A. (1975), Locomotor activity and speed of movements in relation to monoamine-acting drugs. Int. J. Neurol. *10*, 80—98.
12. Herz, A., Zieglgänsberger, W. (1968), The influence of microelectrophoretically applied biogenic amines, cholinomimetics and procaine on synaptic excitation in the corpus striatum. Int. J. Neuropharmakol. *7*, 221—230.
13. Hökfelt, T., Ungerstedt, U. (1969), Electron and fluorescence microscopical studies on the nucleus caudatus and putamen of the rat after unilateral lesions of ascending nigro-neostriatal dopamine neurons. Acta physiol. scand. *76*, 415—426.
14. Hull, C. D., Bernardi, G., Buchwald, N. A. (1970), Intracellular responses of caudate neurons to brain stem stimulation. Brain Res. *22*, 163—179.
15. Hull, C. D., Levine, M. S., Buchwald, N. A., Heller, A., Browning, R. A. (1974), The spontaneous firing pattern of forebrain neurons. I. The effects of dopamine and non—dopamine depleting lesions on caudate unit firing patterns. Brain Res. *73*, 241—262.

16. Kataoka, K., Bak, I. J., Hassler, R., Kim, J. S., Wagner, A. (1974), L-glutamate decarboxylase and choline acetyltransferase activity in the Substantia Nigra and the striatum after surgical interruption of the strio-nigral fibres of the Baboon. Brain Res. *19*, 217—227.

17. Kemp, J. M. (1970), The termination of strio-pallidal and strio-nigral fibres. Brain Res. *17*, 125—128.

18. Kemp, J. M., Powell, T. P. S. (1971), The structure of the caudate nucleus of the cat: Light and electron microscopy. Phil. Trans. R. Soc. Ser. B *262*, 383—401.

19. Kim, J. S., Bak, I. J., Hassler, R., Okada, Y. (1971), Role of Aminobutyric acid (GABA) in the extrapyramidal motor system. II. Some evidence for the existence of a type of GABA-rich strio-nigral neurons. Exp. Brain Res. *14*, 95—104.

20. Kim, J. S. (1973), Effects of 6-hydroxydopamine on acetylcholine and GABA metabolism in rat striatum. Brain Res. *55*, 472—475.

21. Kim, J. S., Hassler, R. (1975), Effects of acute haloperidol on the gamma-aminobutyric system in rat striatum and Substantia Nigra. Brain Res. *88*, 150—153.

22. Kitai, S. T., Wagner, A., Precht, W., Ohno, T. (1975), Nigro-caudate and caudato-nigral relationship: an electrophysiological study. Brain Res. *85*, 44—48.

23. Krnjevic, K. (1974), Some neuroactive compounds in the Substantia Nigra. Advances in Neurology, Vol. 5, pp. 145—153. New York: Raven Press.

24. Mc. Lennan, H., York, D. H. (1967), The action of dopamine on neurones of the caudate nucleus. J. Physiol. (London) *189*, 393—402.

25. Mc. Lennan, H., York, D. H., Cholinergic mechanism in the caudate nucleus. J. Physiol. *187*, 163—175.

26. Maler, L., Fibiger, H. C., Mc. Geer, E. G. (1973), Demonstration of the nigro-striatal projection by silver staining after nigral injections of 6-hydroxydop-amine. Exp. Neurol. *40*, 505—515.

27. Moore, R. Y., Bhatnagan, R. K., Heller, A. (1971), Anatomical and chemical studies of a nigro-neostriatal projection in the cat. Brain Res. *30*, 119—135.

28. Niimi, K., Ikeda, T., Kwamura, S., Inoshita, H. (1970), Efferent projections of the head of the caudate nucleus in the cat. Brain Res. *21*, 327—343.

29. Okada, Y., Hassler, R. (1973), Uptake and release of γ-aminobutyric acid (GABA) in slices of Substantia Nigra of rat. Brain Res. *49*, 214—217.

30. Olivier, A., Parent, A., Simard, H., Poirter, L. J. (1970), Cholinesterasic striatopallidal and striatonigral efferents in the cat and monkey. Brain Res. *18*, 273—282.

31. Precht, W., Yoshida, M. (1971), Blockage of caudate-evoked inhibition of neurons in the Substantia Nigra by picrotoxin. Brain Res. *32*, 229—233.

32. Roberts, E. (1974), γ-aminobutyric acid and nervous system function—a perspective. Biochemical Pharmacology, Vol. 23, pp. 2637—2649. Pergamon Press.

33. Roberts, E. (1974), Disinhibition as an organizing principle in the nervous system. The role of gamma-aminobutyric acid. Advances in Neurology, Vol. 5, pp. 127—144. New York: Raven Press.

34. Svennby, G., Roberts, E. (1973), Bicuculline and N-methylbicuculline-competi-tive inhibitors of brain acetylcholinesterase. J. Neurochem. Vol. *21*, 1025—1026.

35. Szabo, J. (1962), Topical distribution of the striatal efferents in the monkey. Exp. Neurol. *5*, 21—36.
36. Usunoff, K. G., Hassler, R., Wagner, A., Bak, I. J. (1974), The efferent connections of the head of the caudate nucleus in the cat: An experimental morphological study with special reference to a projection to the raphe nuclei. Brain Res. *74*, 143—148.
37. Voneida, T. (1960), An experimental study of the course and destination of fibers arising in the head of the caudate nucleus in the cat and monkey. J. comp. Neurol. *115*, 75—87.
38. Yoshida, M., Precht, W. (1971), Monosynaptic inhibition of neurons of the Substantia Nigra by caudato-nigral fibers. Brain Res. *32*, 225—228.

Authors address: Dr. A. Wagner, Deutschordenstraße 46, D-6000 Frankfurt/ M.-71, Federal Republic of Germany.

Acta Neurochirurgica, Suppl. 24, 199—216 (1977)
© by Springer-Verlag 1977

The Relationship of Hallucinations
to the Depth Structures of the Temporal Lobe*

S. M. Weingarten, D. G. Cherlow, and E. Holmgren

With 10 Figures

Introduction

The purpose of this paper is to present some clinical data which suggests a relationship between abnormal electrical discharges in the depth structures of the temporal lobe and hallucinations. The information has been derived from a series of patients referred to the UCLA Neuropsychiatric Institute who suffered from temporal lobe epilepsy intractable to intensive pharmacologic regimes. The patients were studied with electrodes placed bilaterally in the depth structures of the temporal lobe as well as over the calvarium to monitor the electrical activity of the brain during the ictal and inter-ictal stages. If a unilateral focus for their seizures could be found, it was surgically excised in a second procedure aimed at alleviating their convulsive disorder. One of the patients studied presented initially with a complex hallucination as part of her seizure. In reviewing our series of patients it was of interest to note that hallucinations were produced by electrical stimulation of the depth structures of the temporal lobe in certain patients. The electrical stimulations were carried out in an attempt to induce seizure activity.

A case history and the summarized results of the electrical stimulation studies will be presented to indicate that electrical discharges in the depth structures of the temporal lobe can evoke hallucinatory experiences.

Methods

The patients were placed in a Todd-Wells stereotaxic frame and a ventriculogram carried out through a twist drill made at a predetermined stereotaxic coordinate for the posterior aspect of the right temporal horn as it entered the

* The author wishes to acknowledge the guidance in the surgery and studies undertaken in this series of patients of Dr. Paul H. Crandall, Professor of Neurosurgery, U.C.L.A.

trigonal enlargement of the ventricular system. The ventriculogram was first attempted with air. If the temporal horn was not visualized 3 cc of Convay 90 was mixed with 3 cc saline and injected (Fig. 1). In most cases it was only necessary to fill one temporal horn since the preoperative PEG had demonstrated the symmetry of the ventricular system. Stereotaxic coordinates from the Talairach Atlas [23] were used for electrodes to be inserted into the amygdala, the anterior, mid and posterior portions of the pes hippocampus and hippocampal gyrus. The

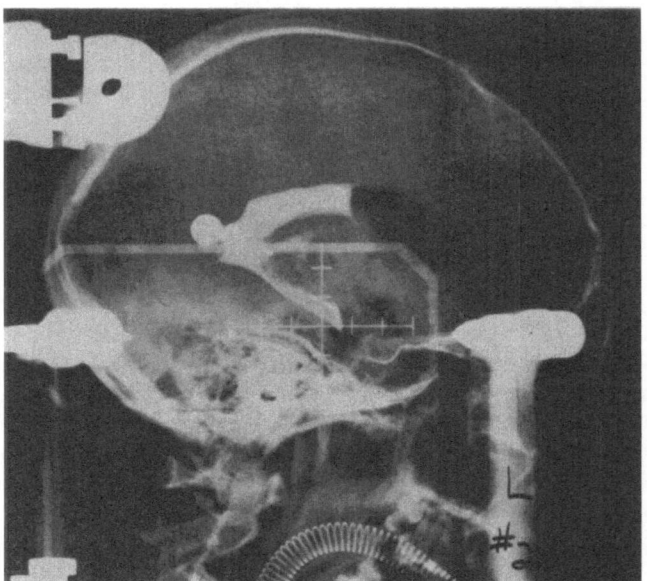

Fig. 1. Ventriculogram

electrodes are placed through hollow screws stereotaxically placed in the calvarium [1] and sealed in position with dental acrylic. The position of the electrodes is confirmed by X-ray (Fig. 2).

The electrodes were either coaxial electrodes or bipolar in type. The coaxial electrodes were stainless steel 25 gauge tubing with 7 mill wire through the center. The diameter of the electrode was 0.021 inch. It was insulated witl epoxylite. The tip was bare for 1 mm and the barrel for 0.5 mm.

The bipolar electrode was a hollow 21 gauge stainless steel tubing with 8 mill wire going down its sides. The electrodes was insulated with epoxylite with the wire bared for 1 mm and the barrel bared for 0.5 mm. Nine microelectrodes of 2 mill platinum alloy could be placed through the hollow core of the bipolar electrodes.

Stimulation sessions lasted several hours and usually took place over two consecutive days. Each of the fourteen electrode sites were tested. A biphasic square pulse from a Grass S-8 stimulator was applied starting at low frequency and voltage. The biphasic pulse were 100 microseconds in duration and were applied in twenty second trains. The number of mamps passing through the electrodes were monitored during stimulation. The resistance of the electrodes varied from 5–12 kOhms. The frequency of stimulation varied from one second to twenty seconds. The voltage ranged from five to thirty volts. The parameters were increased until the patient had a seizure or an afterdischarge or until the current reached a maximum safe level of about 5 mamps. An evoked response was considered to be a change in waveform either to a slow wave, spiking, or both a spike and slow wave which was locked to the stimulation. An afterdischarge was

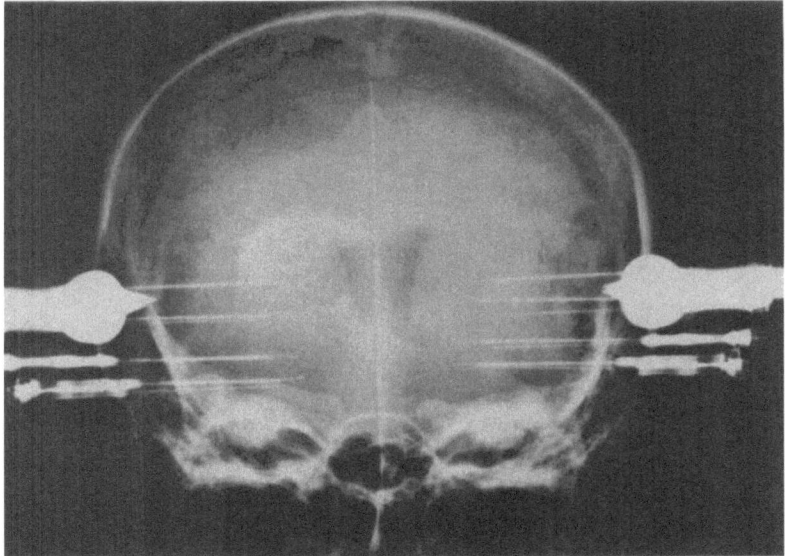

Fig. 2. Depth electrodes in position

an electrical event that continued in a self-perpetuating fashion after the electrical stimulation was terminated.

For each stimulation the parameters of stimulation were monitered and the presence or absence of evoked response, afterdischarge and all subjective and objective clinical effects on the patient were noted.

Case History and Results

A twenty four year old right-handed female was admitted to UCLA in 1971 for evaluation of her seizure disorder. The patient was a product of a caesarean section following thirteen hours of labor but was apparently normal at birth. There was no antenatal illness or trauma. There were no childhood febrile convulsions.

At age sixteen the patient developed dream-like trances which would last thirty seconds and occurred fifteen to thirty times per day. These would occur daily for several weeks and then disappear for several months. The dreams could be pleasant such as seeing a "large cat with a fiddle and a big grin" or be menacing such as a "figure similar to her father shouting and making gestures at her". By age nineteen the patient began to have trance-like states in which she would envision people storming a castle which had a purple color. During these episodes the patient would sit still for a minute out of contact with the environment. By age twenty one the patient's seizures had developed into more typical temporal lobe episodes. She would get a strong feeling of familiarity, a dropping sensation

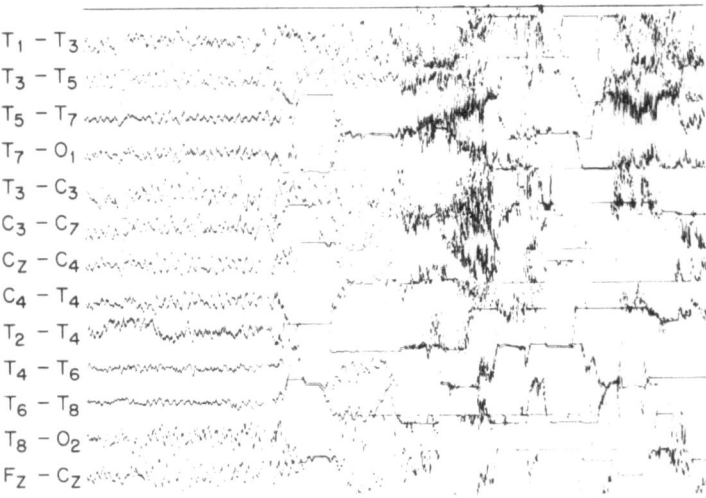

Fig. 3. Seizure—routine EEG

in the pit of her stomach, extreme fear and vertigo; after this aura she appeared to be in an automatism in which she mumbled incoherently, stared straight ahead, licked her lips and looked around. Her left hand almost always rose above her head. If touched during this time she might shy away or become hostile and make defensive gestures. She never fell down or hurt herself. She then had a period of amnesia for three to five minutes. She had no generalized seizures. She had two to three spells per week in spite of multiple medications: Mesantoin, Mysoline and dilantin.

The patient had a B.A. degree. She worked as a secretary although she was having some mild difficulty with recent memory function at work. An arteriogram and PEG done at the Mayo Clinic in 1970 were normal. An EEG showed predominately a right temporal lobe slow wave focus.

The family history was negative for epilepsy. The neurologic examination was normal with the exception that she tended to be somewhat concrete in her interpretation of proverbs.

Prior to the surgical placement of depth electrodes the patient experienced a seizure during a routine EEG (see Fig. 3). There is an abrupt change in the EEG record without any focal EEG signature to localize the origin of the seizure. After depth electrode implantation several seizures were recorded (see Fig. 4). The first change noted in this record is a high frequency low amplitude wave form in the amygdala, right mid pes and right mid gyrus. The high frequency

low amplitude waveform is a rather characteristic antecedent to a seizure discharge and as is seen in this record precedes a build up to a more synchronous
high amplitude discharge involving the right depth structures, spreads to the left
mid gyrus and then there is a diffuse spread of the seizure discharge. Clinically
the seizures had a somewhat stereotyped pattern with the patient sitting up,
mumbling incoherent phrases, fumbling with her hands and having a blank stare
in her eyes. All of the patient's seizures started in the depths of the right temporal

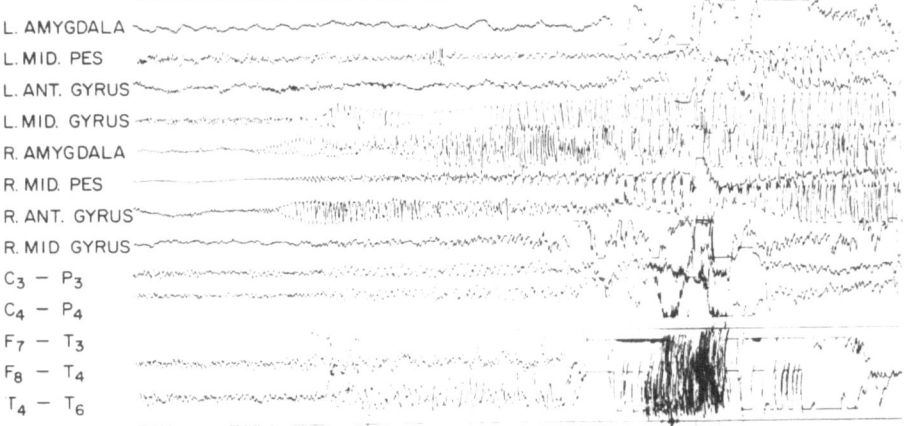

Fig. 4. Seizure—depth EEG

lobe. Occasionally the patient would have seizure-like activity in the depth structures of the right temporal lobe without any spread to other structures (see Fig. 5);
this EEG activity was not associated with any clinical seizure.

During the depth electrode stimulation studies the following dreamlike hallucinations occurred.

Stimulation of the right amygdala with twenty five volts at 1 hz (see Fig. 6)
elicited a diffuse evoked response in the right anterior and mid hippocampus and
hippocampal gyrus. The patient felt that she was back in her bedroom in her
childhood. During a second stimulation in this area she felt that she was in Cambridge, Massachusetts with a date.

Stimulation of the right anterior gyrus with twenty volts at 10 hz set up a
diffuse evoked response in the depth structures of the right temporal lobe (see
Fig. 7) with a moderate afterdischarge in these structures. The patient felt as
though she were having a recurrent dream in which she saw two dogs in her old
house.

Stimulation of the right anterior pes (Fig. 8) activated the right depth structures and the patient felt as though she was standing around the chlorinated
swimming pool of the YWCA as a child.

Stimulation of the right mid pes (Fig. 9) again activated the depth structures
of the right temporal lobe and the patient envisioned an image of an old church,
she then saw the YWCA building and then her old high school.

In stimulating the left anterior gyrus with five volts at 1 hz a response was
elicited in the depth structures of the left side (Fig. 10) and the patient felt that

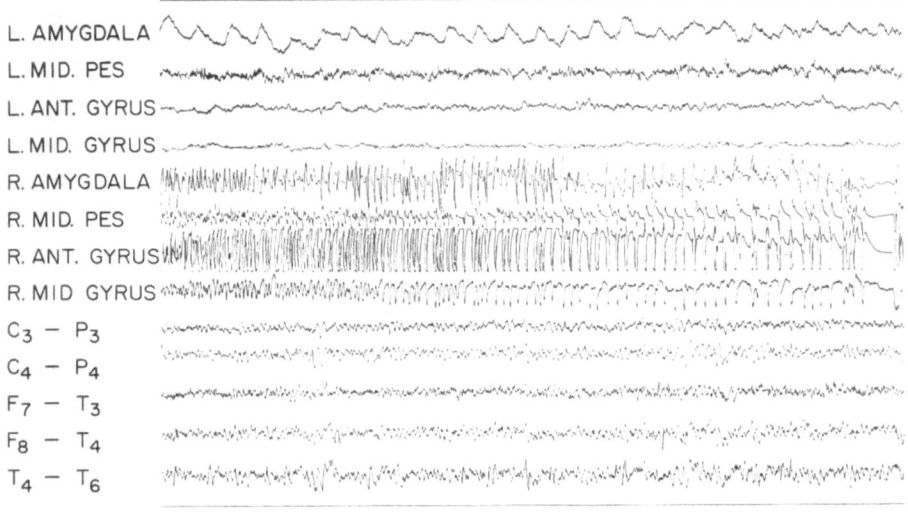

Fig. 5. Sub-clinical seizure—depth EEG

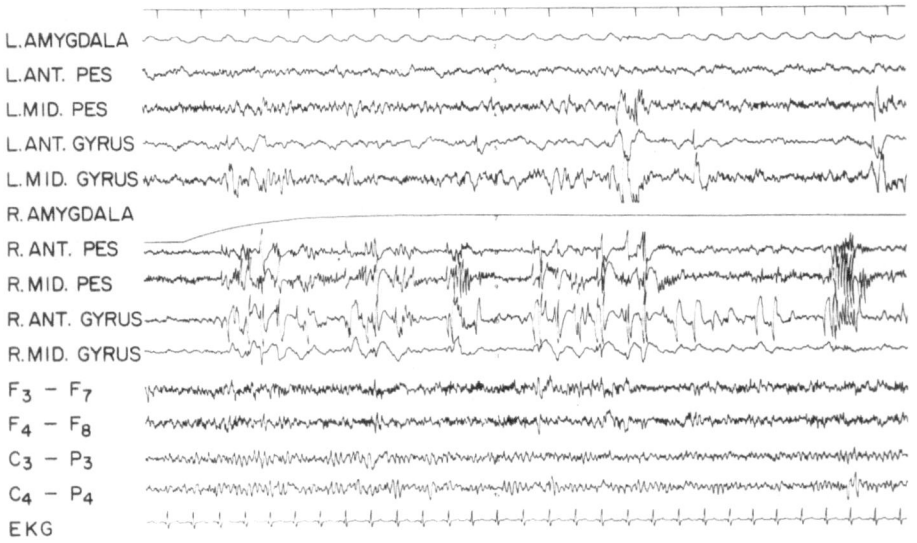

Fig. 6. Stimulation—right amygdala

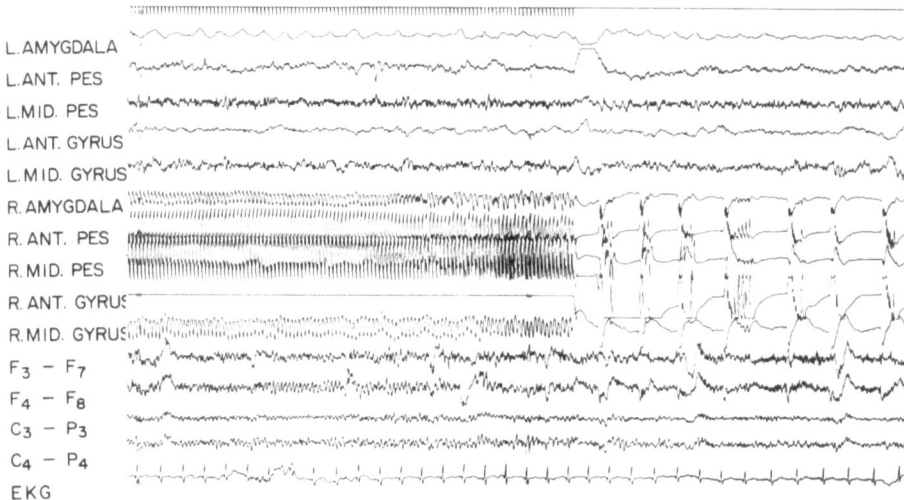

Fig. 7. Stimulation—right anterior gyrus

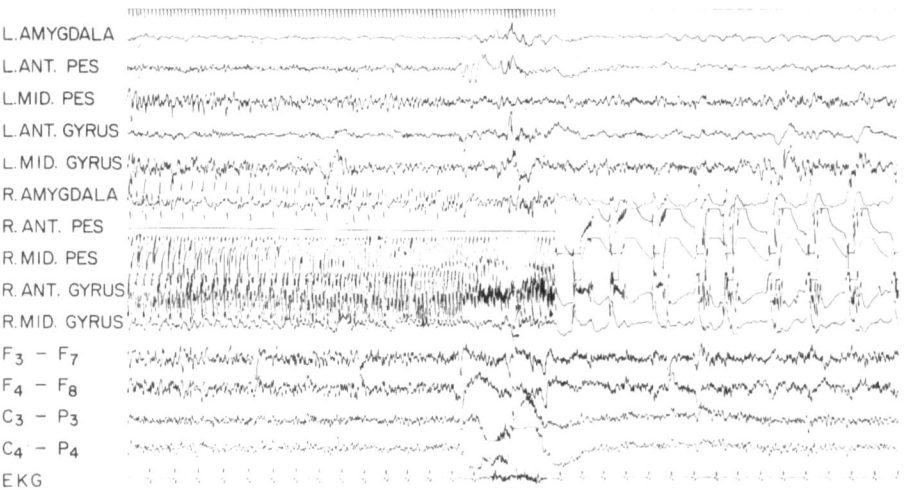

Fig. 8. Stimulation—right anterior pes

she was standing in the backyard of her old house on a lawn between the house
and the badminton court. She could see badminton rackets lying on the ground
with a cover on them. No other stimulations on the left side of the brain in
this patient caused hallucinating activity.

The patient had a right temporal lobectomy in 1971. In the postoperative
period she had a left hemipareses which cleared over a period of one year. She
has not had any seizures or hallucinations since surgery. She has completed a
graduate course in nursing. She works as a nurse, drives a car and has learned
to fly and airplane.

Table 1. *Tingling Sensations in Limbs*

Pt. No.	Site Stimulated	Evoked Response	After Discharge	Site of Pathology	Result
34	LMP	+	0	R	Tingling arms + L leg
32	RAM	+	+	B	Tingling of arms
	RAP	+	+	B	R arm & hand numb
36	LAP	+	+	R	Odd feeling lower limbs
	LAG	+	+	R	Fingers constrictive
	RAM	+	+	R	Legs aching
63	RAM	+	+	R	Feet & legs numb
22	LAP	+	0	R	Tingling legs & back
	RAP	+	+	R	Numbness L leg
	RMG	+	0	R	Sensation R leg
	LAG	0	0	R	Feeling R leg

LAM = Left Amygdala   RAP = Right Anterior Pes
RAM = Right Amygdala   RMP = Right Mid Pes
                         RPP = Right Posterior Pes
LAP = Left Anterior Pes
LMP = Left Mid Pes   R = Right
LPP = Left Posterior Pes   L = Left
                                                B = Bilateral
LAG = Left Anterior Gyrus   RAG = Right Anterior Gyrus
LMG = Left Mid Gyrus   RMG = Right Mid Gyrus
LPG = Left Posterior Gyrus RPG = Right Posterior Gyrus

Because of the interesting responses to depth electrode stimulation
in this patient we reviewed the results of stimulation studies in thirty
nine other patients.

Six patients developed tingling of their limbs (Table 1). The
response varied from ipsilateral to contralateral to bilateral.

Five patients developed sensations over their entire body
(Table 2).

Five patients developed sensations in their head (Table 3).

Fifteen patients developed alimentary sensations (Table 4).

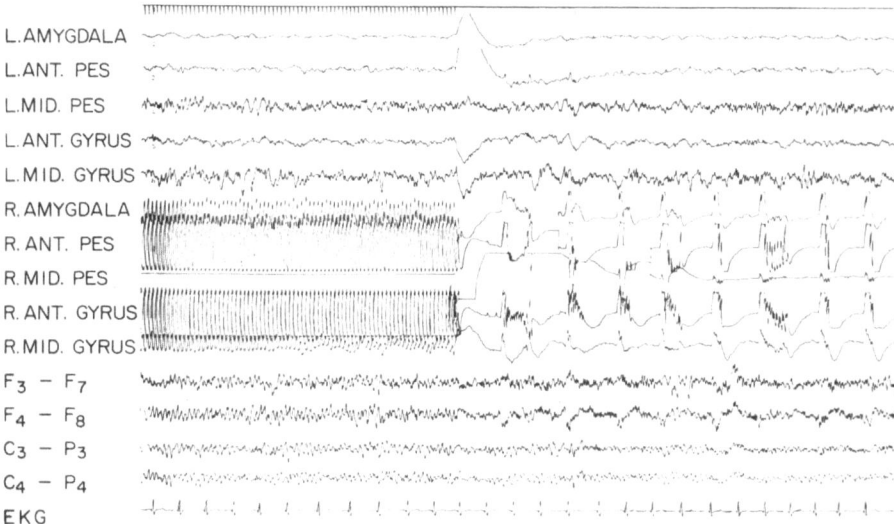

Fig. 9. Stimulation—right mid pes

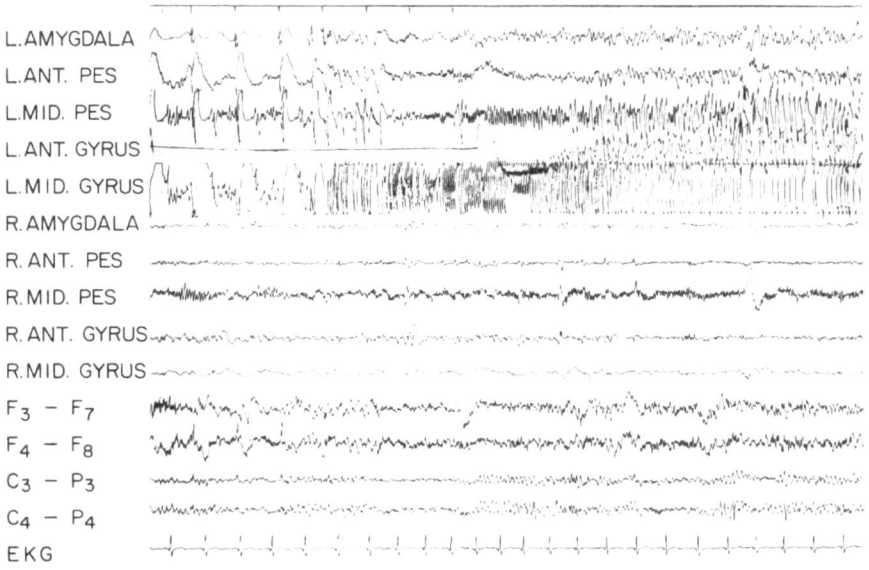

Fig. 10. Stimulation—left anterior gyrus

Eight patients had an emotional response—usually fear—associated with the stimulations (Table 5).

Five patients developed deja vu sensations (Table 6).

Five patients developed dream-like hallucinations (Table 7).

Table 2. *Sensation Over Entire Body*

Pt. No.	Site Stimulated	Evoked Response	After Discharge	Site of Pathology	Result
34	RMP	+	+	R	Tingling all over
	LPP	+	+	R	Tingling all over
57	RAP	+	+	L	Total body sensation
49	RPP	0	0	B	Spinal sensation
	RAP	+	+	B	Total body sensation
63	RAM	+	+	R	Numbness whole body
22	RAM	+	0	R	L side of body & total head

Table 3. *Sensations in Head*

Pt. No.	Site Stimulated	Evoked Response	After Discharge	Site of Pathology	Result
22	LAP	+	+	R	Odd feeling head
	LPG	0	0	R	Odd feeling head
20	RAG	+	0	B	Tingling R side of face
16	RAP	+	0	R	Tight, light feeling head
	LAP	+	+	R	Tight, light feeling head
49	LMP	+ (+ R)	0	R	Funny sensation R side of head
10	LAG	0	0	L	Tingling L side of head

Eight patients developed confusion or amnesia for prolonged periods of time (Table 8). In most of these cases the stimulation either activated bilateral depth structures or was opposite to the side of pathology.

Six patients developed seizures (Table 9). In all of these patients the afterdischarge spread to involve bilateral depth structures.

In this study we were able to find with stimulation of the temporal depth structures similar clinical responses which Penfield found on stimulation of the temporal cortex. In terms of the exact site of stimulation it should be noted that virtually all of the responses were associated with an evoked response with a diffuse involvement of the ipsilateral temporal depth structures. There was a preponderance of these evoked responses with stimulation of the more anterior depth structures of the temporal lobe.

Table 4. *Alimentary Sensation*

Pt. No.	Site Stimulated	Evoked Response	After Discharge	Site of Pathology	Result
38	LAP	+	+	R	Feeling in stomach
49	RAP	+	+	R	Feeling in stomach
53	RAG	+	0	R	Fear in stomach
29	RMG	+	0	L	Sensation throat to stomach
	LAM	+	+	L	Sensation throat to stomach
18	RAP	+	+	R	Epigastric sensation
	RMP	+	+	R	Hollow feeling in stomach
22	RAP	+	+	R	Odd feeling in stomach
	LMP	+	+	R	Odd feeling in stomach
59	LAP	+	+	R	Nausea
34	LMP	+	0	R	Stomach dropped
	RMP	+	+	R	Epigastric sensation
	RAP	+	+	R	Falling feeling in stomach
51	LAM	0	0	R	Strange feeling in stomach
21	LAP	+	0	R	Cold sensation in stomach
16	LAM	+	+	R	Gas in stomach
	LMG	+	+	R	Belch, stomach upset
	RAP	+	+	R	Feeling in stomach
	LAP	+	+	R	Funny feeling in stomach
	LMG	+	+	R	Funny feeling in stomach
62	LMP	+	+	B	Upset stomach
32	RAM	+	0	B	Stomach sick
	RAP	+	+	B	Nausea
	LPP	+	+	B	Nausea
	RAM	+	+	B	Nausea
36	LAG	+	+	R	Nausea
	RAM	+	0	R	Nausea
	RMG	+	+	R	Nausea
55	LAP	+	+	R	Stomachache
	LAG	+	+	R	Stomachache
	RAG	+	+	R	Stomachache

Discussion

The stimulation of the temporal depth structures resulted in tingling sensations in fifteen patients. The subjective response suggests the involvement of a diffuse activation system in that at times the response was ipsilateral, at other times contralateral, and at other times bilateral. The temporal lobe depth structures have been traced

Table 5. *Emotional Response to Stimulation*

Pt. No.	Site Stimulated	Evoked Response	After Discharge	Site of Pathology	Result
34	LAP	+	+	R	Fear
	RMP	+	+	R	Fear
	RAP	+	+	R	Fear
11	RMG	+	+	L	Scared
	RAP	+	+	L	Scared
	RMG	+	+	L	Scared
	LAM	+	+	L	Scared
	LAG	+	+	L	Scared
32	RMP	+	0	B	Sad
	RAM	+	0	B	Angry
13	LAP	+	+	R	Fear
53	LAG	+	+	R	Fear
	RAG	+	0	R	Fear
18	RAG	+	0	R	Tension
30	RAG	+	+	R	Fear
	LAP	+	+	R	Fear
36	RAM	+	0	R	Fear

Table 6. *Déjà Vu*

Pt. No.	Site Stimulated	Evoked Response	After Discharge	Site of Pathology	Result
16	LMG	+	+	R	Déjà vu
62	RAM	+	+	B	Déjà vu
36	RAM	+	+	R	Déjà vu
49	RAM	+	+	B	Déjà vu
	LPG	+	0	B	Déjà vu
	LAP	+	0	B	Déjà vu
	RAP	+	+	B	Déjà vu
53	LAM	+	+	R	Déjà vu

Table 7. *Dream-Like State*

Pt. No.	Site Stimulated	Evoked Response	After Discharge	Site of Pathology	Result
16	LAP	+	+	R	Sees a woman as though in a movie.
	LAM	+	0	R	Feels like he is at White Memorial Hospital & is age 8.
36	LMG	+ +	+ +	R	Feels like a dream.
	LAG	+ +	+ +	R	Hears recitation from Mother Goose rhymes.
49	LMG	+ + +	+	B	Feels like she is watching astronaut on T. V.
	LAG	+ + + +	0	B	Feels like she is in scene in home in her past.
	RAM	+ + +	+	B	"Someone stuck popsicle stick down her throat in Iowa".
	RMP		0	B	Envisions brother's graduation from Valley State.
	RAG	+ +	+ +	B	Lying on a coach.
	RMG	+	+ +	B	Watching a football game.
30	RMG	+ +	+ +	R	Feels like he is a farm tractor. Figures are like in a cartoon.
	LAP	+	+	R	Became scared. Envisioned a game. Not certain what it is.

to the centre median area and the intralaminar group of the thalamus, to the midbrain tegmentum, and to the periaqueductal grey [22, 5, 12]. Penfield related the temporal lobe anatomically to his "centrecephalic system" [20]. Stimulation of the depth structures of the temporal lobe in animals has produced ipsilateral and bilateral motor responses in

Table 8. *Confusion*

Pt. No.	Site Stimulated	Evoked Response	After Discharge	Site of Pathology	Result
11	RMG	+	+	L	Confused
61	L Uncus	+	+	R	Confused
32	LPP	B	B	R	Confused
36	LAG	+	+	R	Confused
	LMG	+	+	R	Confused
	LAP	+	+	R	Confused
38	LAG	+	+	R	Confused
29	RMP	+	+	L	Confused
48	LAP	+	+	R	Confused
30	RMG	B	B	R	Confused

Table 9. *Seizures*

Pt. No.	Site Stimulated	Evoked Response	After Discharge	Site of Pathology	Result
52	LMG	+	B	L	Seizure
13	LAP	+	B	R	Seizure
31	LAG	+	B	R	Seizure
22	RAP	+	+	B	Seizure
68	RAG	B	B	R	Seizure
29	RMP	+	B	L	Seizure

cats and monkeys [16]. The secondary motor and sensory area which is adjacent to and partly overlies the temporal lobe has bilateral representation and is probably involved in temporal lobe automatisms [14]. Anatomical studies [11, 24] have demonstrated the following pathways: 1. The stria terminalis and the amygdalohypothalamic tract are dorsal and ventral connections from the amygdala to the septum and hypothalamus. 2. The inferior thalamic peduncle connects the anterior temporal cortex and amygdala with the dorsomedial and midline thalamic nuclei. 3. The posterior thalamic peduncle connects the anterior temporal region with the pulvinar. 4. The temporopontine tract connects the temporal lobe with the pons. 5. The temporotegmental tract connects the temporal pole, the superior temporal gyrus and the amygdala with the midbrain tegmentum. 6. The fasiculus uncinatus connects basal parts of the frontal lobe to the amygdala and the anterior temporal cortex.

Fifteen patients experienced sensations related to the alimentary system with stimulation of the temporal depth structures. It is of interest in this regard that MacLean [15] documented that gut and respiratory systems are represented in the frontotemporal region in animals by experiments in which strychnine applied in the region of the nucleus solitarius caused spike potentials in the amygdala. In patients he found that the aura of a funny feeling in the stomach was related to discharges in the frontotemporal region.

The most common emotional response to electrical stimulation was fear. Sadness and anger were also elicited. Papez [19] was one of the first to include the temporal depth structures in a system involved with emotional responses. Delgado [2] found the sense of fear to be elicited with stimulation of the amygdala as well as the central grey of the mesencephalon.

Five of our patients experienced deja vu responses with depth electrode stimulation. Higgins [6] also found deja vu responses associated with stimulation of the depth structures of the temporal lobe. He did not find deja vu experiences to be reproduced from stimulation of the temporal cortical structures.

Seven of our patients developed hallucinations of a complex nature associated with stimulation of the depth structures of the temporal lobe. Kubie [12] analyzed the work of Penfield in terms of its implications for psychoanalysis. He described hallucinations as the situation in which the patient perceives himself as somewhere else and yet is aware that he is where he is; he commented that this is the "mental diplopia" referred to by Hughlings Jackson. He indicated that in patients who suffer from psychomotor epilepsy the electrical stimulations of the temporal lobe can reproduce past experiences that have been repressed. He questioned the relationship of the reliving of past experiences with electrical stimulation of the brain to the mechanism of the psychoanalytic process. He postulated that this was Freud's insight in affirming the need to root psychoanalysis securely in biochemistry and neurophysiology.

Kubie was referring to the work of Penfield and Perot [21] in his discussion of hallucinations. Penfield found forty cases out of five hundred twenty eight cases of temporal lobe epilepsy (7.7%) who had hallucinatory experiences with stimulation; fifty three patients experienced ictal hallucinations (10%). He felt that the excitation of the grey matter in the area of the interpretive cortex of the superior temporal gyrus activated mechanisms of recall of past experience. He specifically eliminated the hippocampus and the amygdala as the site of the primary activation of the hallucinatory process. This opinion was later upheld by Jasper and Rasmussen [9]. Penfield did find with stimulation of the temporal neocortex psychical phenomena, sensations in the body, chest and abdomen, occasional senses of taste or small, feelings of deja vu and automatisms. He felt that the automatisms involved the amygdala, but that the deja vu and hallucinations involved primarily the interpretive cortex of the temporal lobe. In reviewing his cases, however, nine of the forty cases stimulated were actually stimulated with electrodes passing into the depth of the temporal lobe in an area seeming to be periamygdaloid in location judging from the description in his paper [21]. He did state that in order for the hallucination to occur it must activate more central grey structures passing from the cortex to the amygdala, to the hippocampus and then into the "centrencephalon".

Horowitz [7] found hallucinations to be elicited from electrical stimulation of the depth structures in ten patients with temporal lobe epilepsy. Ishibashi [8] produced unusual hallucinations in 30% of schizophrenic patients stimulated in depths of temporal lobe. The visual hallucinations were associated with afterdischarges in the depth of the ipsilateral temporal lobe.

MacLean [13] points out that the hypothalamus is the head ganglion of the autonomic nervous system and that as such it was felt to be the center for experiencing and expressing emotion. He indicated, however, that just as the thalamus only participates in a crude way in the awareness of somesthetic sensation but requires the neocortex for fine interpretation that the hypothalamus requires the cortex of the limbic system for the fine appreciation of emotion. He referred to the fact that the temporal lobe and the orbital surface of the frontal lobe have strong connections with the hypothalamus. He felt that the hippocampus was the main afferent receptor for stimuli which eventually effects the hypothalamus.

Douglas [3] felt that the hippocampus excluded stimulation patterns from attention by a process of gating. He felt that the amygdala enhances all incoming stimuli. Stimulation of the amygdala and hippocampus does produce evoked response in the midbrain tegmentum. Both Douglas [3] and Spencer [22] state that the theta wave activity of the hippocampus may be due to recurrent inhibition with Renshau-like cells looping back to the pyramidal cells of the hippocampus. This inhibiting feedback loop is mediated by acetylcholine and blocked with atropine. Votow [24] demonstrated in monkeys that the hippocampus acted to inhibit rage and that its removal lowered the rage threshold.

Kaada [10] also noted the relationship of the temporal lobe depth structures with the reticular system. He further pointed out that the hippocampus, fornix, mammillary bodies, mammillothalamic tract and limbic gyrus all reach the highest development in man; in the brains of vertebrate below mammals there is no medial mammillary nucleus, mammillothalamic tract or anterior nucleus of the thalamus. He felt that this indicated that these structures were not concerned with physiologic activities of a primitive type, but were related to the higher order of emotional and intellectual functions of primates.

Penfield [21] concluded that there was within the brain a remarkable record of stream of consciousness and that stimulation of the temporal neocortex activates it. Mahl [17] found that electrical stimulation of the epileptogenic temporal lobe may produce hallucinations which depended not only on the patient's past experience but his pre-ictal state of mind. Our work and that of Horowitz [7] and Ishibashi [8] indicates that the bodily sensations, alimentary sensations, sense of fear, deja vu experiences and the psychical illusions or hallucinations elicited by Penfield with electrical stimulation of the temporal lobe cortex can all be reproduced by electrical stimulation of the depth structures of the temporal lobe.

References

1. Crandall, P. H., Walter, R. D., Rand, R. W. (1963), Clinical applications on stereotaxically implanted electrodes in temporal lobe epilepsy. J. Neurosurg. 20, 827—840.
2. Delgado, J. M. R., Rosvald, H. E., Looney, E. (1956), Evoking conditioned fear by electrical stimulation of subcortical structures in the monkey brain. J. Comp. Physiol. Psychol. 49, 373—380.
3. Douglas, R. J. (1967), The hippocampus and behaviour. 67, #6, 416—442.
4. Feindell, W., Penfield, W. (1954), Localization of discharge in temporal lobe automatism. AMA Arch. Neurol. Psych. 72, 605—630.
5. Feldman, S. (1962), Neurophysiological mechanism modifying afferent hypothalamus-hippocampal conduction. Exper. Neurol. 5, 269—291.
6. Higgins, J. W., Mahl, G. F., Delgado, M. J. R., Hamlin, H. (1956), Behavioural changes during intracerebral electrical stimulation. AMA Arch. Neurol. Psych. 76, 299—449.
7. Horowitz, M. D., Adams, J. E. (1970), Hallucination on brain stimulation: Evidences for revision of the Penfield hypothesis. In: Origin and mechanisms of hallucination (Keup, W., ed.), pp. 13—22. New York: Plenum Press.
8. Ishibashi, T., Horo, H., Endo, K., Sato, T. (1964), Hallucinations produced by electrical stimulation of temporal lobes in schizophrenic patients. Tohoku J. exp. Med. 82, 124—139.

9. Jasper, H. H., Rasmussen, T. (1958), Studies of clinical and electrical responses to deep temporal stimulation in man with some consideration of functional anatomy. Ass. Res. Nerv. Ment. Dis. *36*, 316—334.
10. Kaada, B. R. (1952), Somatomotor autonomic and EEG responses to electrical stimulation of rhinencephalen and other structures in primates, cats and dogs. Acta Physiol. Scand. *24* (Suppl. 83), 1—263.
11. Klinger, J., Gloor, P. (1960), The connections of the amygdala and of the anterior temporal cortex in the human brain. J. Comp. Neurol. *115*, 333—354.
12. Kubie, L. (1953), Some implications for psychoanalytic analysis of modern concepts of the organization of the brain. Psychoanalytic Quart. *22*, 21—68.
13. MacLean, P. D. (1949), Psychosomatic disease and the visceral brain. Psychosomatic Med. *11*, 338—351.
14. MacLean, P. D. (1950), Developments in EEG: The basal and temporal regions. Yale J. Biol. and Med. *22*, 437—451.
15. MacLean, P. D. (1952), Some psychiatric implications of physiologic studies of frontotemporal portion of limbic system. EEG and Clin. Neurophysiol. *4*, 407—418.
16. MacLean, P. D., Delgado, J. M. R. (1953), Electrical and chemical stimulation of frontotemporal portion of limbic system in the walking animal. EEG and Clin. Neurophysiol. *5*, 91—100.
17. Mahl, G. F., Rothenberg, A., Delgado, J. M. R., Hamlin, H. (1964), Psychological response in human to intracerebral stimulation. Psychosomatic Med. *26*, 337—368.
18. Marsan, C. A., Stoll, J. (1951), Subcortical connections of temporal pole in relation to temporal lobe seizures. AMA Arch. Neurol. Psychiat. *66*, 669—686.
19. Papez, J. W. (1937), A proposed mechanism of emotion. Arch. Neurol. Psychiat. *38*, 725—743.
20. Penfield, W. (1952), Memory mechanism. AMA Arch. Neurol. Psychiat. *66*, 669—686.
21. Penfield, W., Perot, P. (1963), The brain's record of auditory and visual experience. Brain *86*, 595—696.
22. Spencer, W. A., Kandel, E. R. (1961), Hippocampal neuron response to selective actovation of recurrent collaterals of hippocampal axons. Exp. Neurol. *4*, 149—161.
23. Talairach, J., David, M., Tournoux, P. (1958), L'exploration chirurgicale stereotaxique du lobe temporal dans l'epilepsie temporale, p. 136. Paris: Masson et Cie.
24. Votow, C. L. (1960), Certain functional and anatomical relations of the cornu ammonis of the Macaque Monkey. J. Comp. Neurol. *114*, 283—293.
25. Whittock, D. G., Nauta, W. J. (1956), Subcortical projections from the temporal neocortex in Macaca Mulatta. J. Comp. Neurol. *106*, 183—212.

Authors' address: S. M. Weingarten, M.D., Neurological Surgery, 9735 Wilshire Boulevard, Beverly Hills, CA 90212, U.S.A.

Section IV

Pain

Abstracts of the papers of the combined scientific session of IV World Congress of Psychiatric Surgery and II Meeting of the European Society for Stereotactic and Functional Neurosurgery. The full texts will be published in the Proceedings of the IV World Congress of Psychiatric Surgery.

Acta Neurochirurgica, Suppl. 24, 219 (1977)

Research Laboratory of Clinical Stereotaxy VUHB, Neurosurgical Clinic,
Bratislava, Czechoslovakia

Observation of Kindling Phenomenon in Treatment of the Pain by Means of Stimulation in Thalamus

M. Šramka, P. Sedlák, and P. Nádvorník

The results of pain treatment by means of stimulation of the spinal cord structures particularly dorsal column stimulation encourages stimulation of deep brain structures.

We stimulated 4 patients in the thalamus. An unusual complication occurred in one patient. In a female patient suffering from phantom pain of upper right extremity the electrodes were introduced into DM, VCP and CM thalami and the stimulation was carried out for three weeks. The stimulation was then interrupted because of minor jerks, which we originally considered to be neodyskinesis known as a complication in stereotactic treatment of Parkinsonism. Within a few days, however, the jerks intensified, changed into Jackson paroxysms and, finally, into epileptic attacks of the grand mal type.

The iatrogenic epilepsy fortunately was cured by anticonvulsant. In EEG record the attacks exhibited a marked EEG correlate.

This complication may be compared to kindling phenomenon of Goddard described in experimental animals.

Authors' address: Šramka, M., M.D., Ph.D., Research Laboratory of Clinical Stereotaxy VUHB, 809 46 Bratislava, Czechoslovakia.

Acta Neurochirurgica, Suppl. 24, 221 (1977)

Servicio de Neurocirugía, Fundación Jimenez Diaz, Madrid, Spain

Electroanalgesia: Stimulation at Different Levels of the Nervous System

J. Burzaco

Since 1971 we have been using the electro-stimulation method to relieve drug-resistant, chronic pain. Different shaped electrodes have been placed at four levels of the nervous system: peripheral nerves, Gasserian ganglion, spinal cord and thalamus. The receiver is located in the subcutaneous tissue of the anterior thoracic wall.

The method has been used in 25 patients, during a 4 years period, while as many other patients have been treated by the more classical procedures: cordotomy and stereotactic thalamotomy. The reasons for selecting one or other type of treatment is presented.

A theory for the optimal placement of the electrodes for thalamic stimulation is presented and the main technical problems of this surgery, its complications and results. At present we should keep in mind that two important links of the complex chain of events involved in the phenomenon of pain are out of control in the electrical stimulation method: firstly, there is a significant change of energy when the electric stimulus is transferred to a nerve impulse. And finally, the nerve impulse is on transformed in painful sensation. Despite its limitations, the electroanalgesic method has a firm place in the treatment of drug resistant, invaliding pain.

Author's address: Dr. J. Burzaco, Servicio de Neurocirugía, Fundación Jimenez Diaz, Madrid, Spain.

Acta Neurochirurgica, Suppl, 24, 223–225 (1977)
© by Springer-Verlag 1977

Department of Neurosurgery, University Central Hospital, Helsinki, Finland

Anterior Pulvinotomy in the Treatment of Intractable Pain

L. Laitinen

Between 1970 and 1974, I carried out stereotactic anterior pulvinotomy on 41 patients suffering from intractable pain. The series was selected; we tried to exclude patients with hysterical and/or depressive symptoms. Ten patients suffered from phantom limb pain, 10 from thalamic pain, 6 from peripheral neuralgia, 5 from cancer pain, 5 from zoster neuralgia and 5 from anaesthesia dolorosa. Twenty-two were men and 19 women. Their ages ranged from 32 to 74 years, with an average of 56 years. Duration of pain ranged from 3 months to 26 years, with an average of 6,5 years. Most of the patients had received large doses of analgesics, psychotherapy, hypnotic therapy and accupuncture without long-lasting effect.

I used my own stereotactic instrument. The frontal horn was cannulated through a frontal burr hole, 10 ml of CSF was withdrawn, and 25 ml of air was insufflated, which gave a good visualization of the third ventricle. The pulvinar target lay 3 mm behind the rostral margin of the posterior commissure and 5 mm above the continued intercommissural line. Twenty-one patients had medial pulvinotomy, where the target lay 10–11 mm lateral to the midline. The thermocoagulation lesion was presumed to be 5–6 mm in diameter. In addition to the medial lesion 20 patients had another lesion in the lateral part of the nucleus, 15–16 mm from the midline. This second lesion was as large as the medial one, and we assume that the two fused into a single lesion which destroyed the whole anterior pulvinar.

Two patients with bilateral pain underwent bilateral medial pulvinotomy in one session; in 39 cases the operation was unilateral and contralateral to the side of pain. All operations were done under local anaesthesia with premedication consisting of 50 mg cyclizine lactate (Marzine®). Physiological and psychological tests were made during surgery. In 23 of the 41 patients the lateral ventricles were dilated; usually the ventricle of the pulvinotomy side was wider than the other.

The immediate effect of pulvinotomy was often good: 19 of the 41 patients were completely without pain and needed no analgesics postoperatively. Twelve reported some relief of pain. They stated that the sharp component of the pain had gone, but there was still some residual slow pain which seldom required analgesics. Ten patients did not obtain any benefit from the operation.

Pulvinotomy caused little stress. After surgery none of the patients were drowsy or tired, as they so commonly are after ventrolateral thalamotomy. Therefore it is unlikely that the very good immediate effect was caused by dampened psychic activity.

The good immediate effect was, unfortunately, often of short duration. In most patients the pain recurred within a few weeks, but recurrencies sometimes developed more than one year afterwards. Twenty-nine months after surgery, on the average, 12 patients (29%) were still painfree. Two of them had died free from the chronic pain 2 and 13 months, respectively, after pulvinotomy. Eleven patients felt that the operation had had a long-lasting fairly good effect, while 18 (44%) experienced the pain unchanged or worse than ever before.

Medial pulvinotomy seemed to give results as good as the double lesion in the medial and lateral pulvinar.

Side-effects were noticed in 6 patients. An elderly man was confused for 3 days after a medial and lateral lesion for phantom limb pain. Another patient had a feeling of numbness and heaviness in his contralateral thigh. The tendon reflexes were exaggerated but the plantar reflexes were normal. No cutaneous sensory deficit was detected. Two further patients had a similar, although slighter sensation of numbness and hyperactive tendon reflexes on the contralateral side of the body. All 3 patients with this proprioceptive damage had had a double medio-lateral lesion. This side-effect seems to be long-lasting or permanent, and the patients suffer from it considerably. In one patient with peripheral neuralgia after contusions of the brain and pelvis the operation caused transient diplopia. The sixth patient had semantic aphasia after bilateral medial pulvinotomy. Previously, she had had a cancer metastasis in her left parieto-occipital lobe. There was no mortality in this series.

The present study confirms the findings of Richardson (1967), Yoshii (1970), and Yoshii, Kudo, and Shimizu (1973) that anterior pulvinotomy may have a beneficial effect on chronic pain. The immediate effect is often good, but, as so often in pain surgery, there is a tendency for the pain to recur later. so, about 2½ years after pulvinotomy only one fourth of the patients were painfree, while almost half had obtained no long-lasting benefit. Nevertheless, the effect of pulvinotomy seems to be better than that of centre median thalamotomy; of the 32 patients whom I had previously operated on in the centre median, only 2 were painfree 3 years later.

Electrophysiological investigations during these operations showed that the anterior pulvinar has strong connexions with the temporal cortex. I am tempted to suggest that this nucleus normally facilitates the temporal associative cortical areas to classify and interpret sensory input. In chronic pain, this input is changed or completely lacking, the brain is not able to classify the situation, and this failure causes a continuous alarm state. Pulvinotomy may alter this dysfunction transiently or permanently. A similar mechanism may underly the beneficial effect of electrical stimulation of the skin, posterior columns and some sensory pathways in the brain.

In recent years the transcutaneous nerve stimulation method has clearly diminished the need for pulvinotomy. In our efforts to relieve chronic pain, we have abandoned destructive lesions, and are now concentrating on electrical stimulation of the pulvinar through implanted devices.

Author's address: L. Laitinen, M.D., Department of Neurosurgery, Topelius 5, SF-00260 Helsinki 26, Finland.

Acta Neurochirurgica, Suppl. 24, 227 (1977)
© by Springer-Verlag 1977

Institute of Neurosurgery, University of Buenos Aires, Buenos Aires, Argentina

Paraqueductal Mesencephalotomy
for Facial Central Pain

J. R. Schvarcz

Facial central pain is usually difficult to manage. Although stereotactic trigeminal nucleotomy is a valuable procedure, there is still a group of supra-caudalis origin, which is resistant to current techniques. For them, paraqueductal lesions offer an attractive approach.

Five cases are reported with intractable facial pain due to brain stem vascular insults. The target area is the contralateral central gray, parallel to, and at 2 mm of the lateral wall of the aqueduct, at intercollicular level.

Stimulation resulted in a variety of sensory, emotional and autonomic responses. The threshold sensory responses were referred to the centre of the face, generally deep within the oral and nasal cavities. With increased intensity, they spread to the central thoracic and upper abdominal region. Gustatory and visceral sensations were occasionally elicited. A strong emotional reaction was always produced, of a very unpleasant, fearful quality. Autonomic changes, such as blushing, sweating and piloerection, were often induced.

Excellent results were obtained in all but one case. Follow up ranged between 18 and 27 months. Both the hyperpathia and the deep pain were relieved. However, only subjective analgesia was achieved, without demonstrable sensory loss. No other side effect but loss of upward gaze was produced.

Author's address: Dr. J. R. Schvarcz, Las Heras 2012, Buenos Aires 1127, Argentina.

Acta Neurochirurgica, Suppl. 24, 229 (1977)

Department of Functional Neurosurgery and Neuronuclear Medicine, Neurosurgical
University Hospital, Freiburg i. Br., Federal Republic of Germany

Late Results of Central Stereotactic Interventions for Pain

F. Mundinger and P. Becker

The present report deals with the results of 64 central stereotactic pain interventions out of a total of 138 (date: February 1975)
performed since 1952. In the majority of cases we were treating
either phantom pain, stump causalgia, trigeminus neuralgia, the
thalamus syndrom or other chronic pain produced by tabes dorsalis
and others.

We eliminated the basal segments of the ventrocaudal nuclei
(v.c.pc.) and the nucleus limitans with or without the medial
nucleus; in later series we exclusively eliminated the non-specific
thalamic systems (v.c., intralaminary nuclei, lamella medialis, centrum medianum) with or without the additional destruction of the
medial nucleus and the pulvinar.

Out of the 22 interventions of cases of phantom pain and
causalgies all patients were postoperatively improved and $3/5$ free
of pain. 4–6 years later these patients were still free of pain,
$7/10$ improved out of the 18 interventions of patients with intractable
trigeminus neuralgias (for example, after herpes zoster) half of
them were postoperatively pain-free, half of the cases improved
and $3/5$ of them remained so after 1–2 years.

The long-term results for the 17 interventions of patients with
thalamic syndroms showed $4/5$ to have experienced satisfactory-to
good improvement.

Author's address: Prof. Dr. F. Mundinger and Dr. P. Becker, Neurosurgical
University Hospital, Department for Functional Neurosurgery and Neuronuclear
Medicine, Hugstetter Straße 55, D-7800 Freiburg i. Br., Federal Republic of
Germany.

Acta Neurochirurgica, Suppl. 24, 231 (1977)

Department of Neurosurgery, Ciudad Sanitaria Virgen del Rocio, Sevilla, Spain

Stereotactic Cryothalamotomy for Pain

F. Rodriguez-Burgos and V. Arjona

Stereotactic cryothalamotomy was performed in twenty-four patients with severe "intractable" pain. In eighteen patients the pain was due to malignancy. Three patients had "central" pain following traumatic paraplegia, one suffered from anesthesia dolorosa, one had pain consecutive to lung abscess and another one causalgia.

The operations were always done with the patient under local anesthesia. The Leksell stereotactic frame was used and the lesions were made with the Cooper cryogenic system. We aimed to destroy most of the medial-basal thalamus, between the internal medullary lamina and the lateral wall of the third ventricle, affecting mainly CM and parafascicularis nuclei.

Three lesions were usually made in each side at the same operative session, and no complications occurred during operations.

All patients lost their pain during operation or immediately after. In some patients the pain recurred later.

A detailed analysis of the long-term results and complications is made. Indications and implications of this type of surgery are discussed.

Author's address: Dr. F. Rodriguez-Burgos and Dr. V. Arjona, Department of Neurosurgery, Ciudad Sanitaria Virgen del Rocio, Sevilla, Spain.

Acta Neurochirurgica, Suppl. 24, 233 (1977)

Limbic Target Surgery in the Treatment of Intractable Pain With Drug Addiction

M. H. Brown

In the past 20 years limbic target surgery was used in 41 patients for control of intractable pain. Anxiety-depressive states coexisted with pain in most cases and produced strong psychogenic fixation. Most patients had antecedent polysurgery that was ineffective and were dependent on heavy medication. Phantom limb syndrome was included in the series.

Single targets in the anterior cingulum as well as multiple limbic targets were used depending on individual input data. There was no surgical mortality. Case reports and motion picture interviews are presented with a statistical summary of the results.

Author's address: M. Hunter Brown, M.D., Santa Monica Boulevard 2021, Santa Monica, CA 90404, U.S.A.

Acta Neurochirurgica, Suppl. 24, 235 (1977)

Neurosurgical Clinic Steglitz of the Free University of Berlin

Advantage and Limits of Intracerebral Pain Stereotaxy

G. Bouchard, Y. Mayanagi, and L. F. Martins

An evaluation is given of the results of 60 patients treated stereotactically for unbearable pain within the last 7 years. These operations, most important in the management of pain in malignant diseases, proved to have minimal risks (no operative death) and few complications. 51 had malignant diseases. 4 anesthesia dolorosa following trigeminal surgery, another 3 thalamic pain following cerebro-vascular diseases and the remaining 2 phantom pain. Combined methods, in use since 1966, *e.g.*, coagulation within centre median, porta thalami and anterior dorsomedial nuclei or centre med.-parafascicularis-limitans and pulvinar with medial dorsomedial nuclei in one or both hemisphere are compared in different groups (malignancies situated 1. in the head and neck, 2. in the upper and 3. in the lower half of the body). Those results together with the results in non-malignant pain syndromes underwent critical evaluation of the operative stereotactic procedure. A proven pain reducing effect was found when we included a pulvinar coagulation. Besides malignant processes anesthesia dolorosa and thalamic pain respond well. Phantom limb pain, however so far had no relief after cerebral stereotactic intervention. The operative technique, intraoperative electrophysiological research and post mortem histological verifications are reported.

Authors' address: Dr. med. G. Bouchard, Nervenarzt, Neurochirurg, Friedrich-Ebert-Straße 77, D-3500 Kassel, Federal Republic of Germany.